X. Rogiers ■ H. Bismuth ■ R.W. Busuttil ■ D.C. Broering ■ D. Azoulay ■ (Eds.)

Split liver transplantation

Theoretical and practical aspects

X. Rogiers
H. Bismuth
R. W. Busuttil
D. C. Broering
D. Azoulay
(Eds.)

Split liver transplantation

Theoretical and practical aspects

With 55 figures
in 76 separate illustrations
and 20 tables

STEINKOPFF
DARMSTADT

Springer

Xavier Rogiers, MD
Universitätsklinikum
Hamburg-Eppendorf
Abt. für Hepatobiliäre Chirurgie
Martinistraße 52
20246 Hamburg, Germany

Dieter C. Broering, MD
Universitätsklinikum
Hamburg-Eppendorf
Abt. für Hepatobiliäre Chirurgie
Martinistraße 52
20246 Hamburg, Germany

Henri Bismuth, MD
Hôpital Paul Brousse
12, av. Paul Vaillant Couturier
94804 Villejuif Cedex, France

Daniel Azoulay, MD
Hôpital Paul Brousse
Departement of Hepatobiliary
Surgery
14, av. Paul Vaillant Couturier
94850 Villejuif Cedex, France

Ronald W. Busuttil, MD
University of California
Los Angeles
Transplant Center
Department of Surgery
10833 LeConte Ave.
Los Angeles, CA 90024, USA

ISBN 978-3-7985-1256-6 ISBN 978-3-642-57523-5 (eBook)
DOI 10.1007/978-3-642-57523-5

Die Deutsche Bibliothek – CIP-Einheitsaufnahme
A catalogue record for this publication is available from Die Deutsche Bibliothek

http://www.steinkopff.springer.de

Originally published by Steinkopff-Verlag Darmstadt in 2002

Production: Klemens Schwind
Cover Design: Erich Kirchner, Heidelberg
Typesetting: K+V Fotosatz GmbH, Beerfelden

SPIN 10782735 105/7231-5 4 3 2 1 0 – Printed on acid-free paper

Preface

The last decade has seen an explosion in the surgical efforts to overcome the shortage of liver grafts for transplantation. The end of the 1990s saw the development of the concepts of reduced, split and living donor transplantation by the transplant pioneers and their first applications in practice. During the 1990s many centers throughout the world invested their experience to further develop this into safe and teachable standardized procedures with excellent results. The result of this development is not only that split liver transplantation between adults and children became a validated surgical technique, but also the real possibility of achieving 0% mortality for children on the waiting list today.

However, like many new surgical techniques, its success does not only depend on adequate patient selection (in this case selection of the donor and the recipients!), but also on the avoidance of mistakes that were already experienced by previous surgeons. It is this principle, combined with the need of spreading split liver transplantation knowledge, that led to the organization of the first practical split liver transplantation course in Hamburg in March 2000.

Writing about the surgeon scientist, Joseph E. Murray described one of the differences between the scientist and surgeon: "*The scientist can wait for all the data to become available whereas the surgeon must make a decision based on available data.*" This book aims to provide the surgeon, who wants to start split liver transplantation with the data available today.

Experienced transplant surgeons, who taught in the course, present different aspects of split liver transplantation from surgical anatomy to technical performance, from donor and recipient selection to the organizational aspect, from historical aspects to future visions!

We hope that this book may contribute to the propagation of the split liver technique and may encourage research to develop split liver transplantation for two adult patients.

Hamburg, June 2002 XAVIER ROGIERS

List of contents

1 | History, status quo and logistics

2 | Anatomy

3 | Techniques for splitting the liver

4 | The recipient

5 | Results and outlook

List of contributors

FARIN AMERSI, MD
University of California
Los Angeles
Transplant Center
Department of Surgery
10833 LeConte Ave.
Los Angeles, CA 90024, USA

DANIEL AZOULAY, MD
Hôpital Paul Brousse
Departement of Hepatobiliary
Surgery
14, av. Paul Vaillant Couturier
94850 Villejuif Cedex, France

JAQUES BELGHITI, MD
Hôpital Beaujon
100, bd. du Général-Leclerc
92118 Clichy Cedex, France

HENRI BISMUTH, MD
Hôpital Paul Brousse
12, av. Paul Vaillant Couturier
94804 Villejuif Cedex, France

DIETER C. BROERING, MD
Universitätsklinikum
Hamburg-Eppendorf
Abteilung für Hepatobiliäre
Chirurgie
Martinistraße 52
20246 Hamburg, Germany

RONALD W. BUSUTTIL, MD
University of California
Los Angeles
Transplant Center
Department of Surgery
10833 LeConte Ave.
Los Angeles, CA 90024, USA

DENIS CASTAING, MD
Hôpital Paul Brousse
Departement of Hepatobiliary
Surgery
14, av. Paul Vaillant Couturier
94800 Villejuif Cedex, France

JEAN DE VILLE DE GOYET, MD
Birmingham Children's Hospital
Steelhouse Lane
Birmingham B46NH
United Kingdom

GUISEPPE M. ETTORE, MD
Hôpital Beaujon
100, bd. du Général-Leclerc
92118 Clichy Cedex, France

OLIVIER FARGES, MD
Hôpital Beaujon
100, bd. du Général-Leclerc
92118 Clichy Cedex, France

RASHID M. GHOBRIAL, MD
University of California
Los Angeles
Transplant Center
Department of Surgery
10833 LeConte Ave.
Los Angeles, CA 90024, USA

BRUNO GRIDELLI, MD
Ospedali Riuniti
Department of Pediatric Liver
Transplantation
Largo Barozzi 1
24100 Bergamo, Italy

MATTHIAS GUNDLACH, MD
Klinik für Allgemein-,
Visceral- und Thoraxchirurgie
Klinikum Duisburg
Wedaukliniken
Zu den Rethwesen 9
47055 Duisburg, Germany

CHRISTIAN HILLERT, MD
Universitätsklinikum
Hamburg-Eppendorf
Abteilung für Hepatobiliäre
Chirurgie
Martinistraße 52
20246 Hamburg, Germany

TOM KARBE
Universitätsklinikum
Hamburg-Eppendorf
Abteilung für Hepatobiliäre
Chirurgie
Martinistraße 52
20246 Hamburg, Germany

GEERT KAZEMIER, MD
Hospital Erasmus
Medical Clinic
Dr. Molewaterplain 40
3015 GD Rotterdam
The Netherlands

TETSUJA KIUCHI, MD
Kyoto University Hospital
Department of Transplant
Surgery
54, Kawara-Kyoto, Shogoin
Sakyo-Ku Kyoto 606-8507, Japan

ALFRED KOENIGSRAINER, MD
Universität Innsbruck
Klinische Abteilung für
Transplantations-Chirurgie
Anichstraße 35
6020 Innsbruck, Austria

ROBERT KUETEMEIER
Universitätsklinikum
Hamburg-Eppendorf
Abteilung für Hepatobiliäre
Chirurgie
Martinistraße 52
20246 Hamburg, Germany

RUTH LADURNER, MD
Universitätsklinik für Chirurgie
Anichstraße 35
6020 Innsbruck, Austria

JOHAN F. LANGE, MD
Hospital Erasmus
Medical Clinic
Dr. Molewaterplain 40
3015 GD Rotterdam
The Netherlands

REIMUND MARGREITER, MD
Universitätsklinik für Chirurgie
Anichstraße 35
6020 Innsbruck, Austria

GUILLERMO
MARIN-HARGREAVES, MD
Hôpital Paul Brousse
15, av. Paul Vaillant Couturier
94850 Villejuif Cedex, France

JEAN-BERNARD OTTE, MD
Université Catholique de Louvain
Cliniques Universitaires Saint-Luc
Avenue Hippocrate
10 UCL 10/1401
1200 Brussels, Belgium

Jorge Reyes, MD
University of Pittsburgh
Department Transplant Surgery
4th Fl. Falk Clinic
3601 Fifth Ave
Pittsburgh, PA L5238, USA

Xavier Rogiers, MD
Universitätsklinikum
Hamburg-Eppendorf
Abteilung für Hepatobiliäre
Chirurgie
Martinistraße 52
20246 Hamburg, Germany

Alain Sauvanet, MD
Hôpital Beaujon
100, bd. du Général-Leclerc
92118 Clichy Cedex, France

Hans J. Schlitt, MD
Medizinische Hochschule
Hannover
Klinik für Viszeral- und
Transplant-Chirurgie
Carl Neubergstraße 1
30623 Hannover, Germany

Jan Schulte am Esch, MD
Universitätsklinikum
Hamburg-Eppendorf
Abteilung für Hepatobiliäre
Chirurgie
Martinistraße 52
20246 Hamburg, Germany

Egbert Sieders, MD
Hepatobiliary Surgery
Academisch Ziekenhuis
Groningen
P.O. Box 30001
9700 RH Groningen
The Netherlands

Martin J.H. Slooff, MD
Hepatobiliary Surgery
Academisch Ziekenhuis
Groningen
P.O. Box 30001
9700 RH Groningen
The Netherlands

Daniel Sommacale, MD
Hôpital Beaujon
100, bd. du Général-Leclerc
92118 Clichy Cedex, France

Koichi Tanaka, MD
Kyoto University Hospital
Department of Transplantation
and Immunology
54, Kawara-Kyoto, Shogoin
Sakyo-Ku Kyoto 606-8507, Japan

Stefan Topp, MD
Universitätsklinikum
Hamburg-Eppendorf
Abteilung für Hepatobiliäre
Chirurgie
Martinistraße 52
20246 Hamburg, Germany

Hassan Yersiz, MD
University of California
Los Angeles
Transplant Center
Department of Surgery
10833 LeConte Ave.
Los Angeles, CA 90024, USA

1 History, status quo and logistics

1.1 J.-B. Otte

History of split liver transplantation

■ Introduction

We have reviewed published work regarding first attempts of *ex situ* split liver transplantation, the main European and American centers series of *ex situ* and *in situ* split, our own experience, the data collected (1990–1993) by the European Split Liver Transplantation Registry, as well as all data collected between 1988 and June 30, 1999 by the European Liver Transplant Registry.

■ First attempts of *ex situ* split

Four cases were performed between February and November 1988 (Table 1), three in Europe (Hannover, Villejuif, Brussels) [1–3] and one in Chicago, USA (4). Two livers were split along the umbilical scissure and shared between one adult (right split graft) and one child (left split graft). The remaining two livers were split along the main scissure and shared between two adult recipients or two pediatric recipients (graft procured from a pediatric donor). Seven of the 10 recipients were at high risk. Three patients (2 children, 1 adult) survived and are currently alive (≥12 years).

■ Main European single – center series of *ex situ* split

Collectively, there were 202 recipients comprising 97 adults and 105 children (Tables 2 and 3). The percentage of high-risk patients ranged between 12% and 75%. The overall patient survival rate ranged between 75% and 93%; overall graft survival rate ranged between 67% and 83%. Incidence of surgical complications is recorded in Table 3. Primary non-function was unusual. The incidence of vascular thrombosis was not different from full size liver transplantation whereas the incidence of biliary complications (mainly leaks from missed radicles or cut surfaces and ischemic-like strictures) was likely more elevated.

Table 1. First attempts of *ex situ* split

Center	Date	Report	Recipients	Outcome Function-survival	Plane of partition
Hannover Pichlmay [1]	Feb. 88	1988	L: 2 y-BA R: 63 y-PBC	ReTX-4 mo-dead AW 12 yrs	Umbilical scissure
Paul-Brousse Bismuth [2]	May 88	1989	L: 45 y-ALF-ICU	Recovered from coma Died POD 20, MOF sepsis	Main scissure
			R: 55 y-ALF-ICU	Regained nl liver function Died POOD 45, CMV disease	
Chicago Broelsch [4]	July 88	1990	L: 3 mo-subac.-ICU R: 7 mo α-1 ATD	Died POD 2, heart failure AW 12 yrs	Main scissure
Brussels Otte [3]	Nov. 88	1990	L: 5 y Tyrosinemia-Hosp.	AW 12 yrs	Umbilical scissure
			R: 55 y-Endstage cirrhosis Chronic rej. renal Tx (combined L-K)	Died POD 3, sepsis candida	

L left split graft; *R* right split graft; *BA* biliary atresia; *PCB* primary biliary cirrhosis; *ALF* acute liver failure; *ICU* intensive care unit; *α-1 ATD* α-1 antitrypsine deficiency; *POD* postoperative day

Table 2. Main European single-center series of *ex situ* split

	n	Adults	Children	% high risk	Patient survival (%)			Graft survival (%)		
					Ad	Ch	Overall	Ad	Ch	Overall
Paul-Brousse (95) [5]	27	26	1	22			79			78
King's College (88–96) [6]	41	15	26	12			90			88
Cochin, Paris [7]	16	6	10	75			75			69
Brussels (88–99)	53	23	30	28	83	83	83	73	77	75
Birmingham (92–96) [8]	23	9	14	58	77	78	78			67
Birmingham (98–00) [9]	42	18	24		89	96	93	78	88	83

Ad adult; *Ch* children

Table 3. Main European single-center series of *ex situ* split. Percent complications

	n	Bleeding	PNF	Arterial thromb.	Portal thromb.	Biliary	Venous outflow obstruction
Paul-Brousse (95) [5]	27	4	4	15	0	22	–
King's College (88–96) [6]	41	5	0	2	0	14	–
Cochin, Paris [7]	16	12	0	25	12	25	
Brussels (84–99)	63	2	6	3	–	19	2
Birmingham (92–96) [8]	24	8	4	4	0	12	0
Birmingham (98–00) [9]	42		–	5	0	14	2

Table 4. Main American single-center series of *ex situ* split

	n	Adults	Children	% high risk	Patient survival (%)			Graft survival (%)		
					Ad	Ch	Overall	Ad	Ch	Overall
Chicago (88–90) [10]	30	5	25	26	20	67	50	20	48	43
Omaha (88–91) [11]	10	1	9	73			69			67
Madison (94–95) [12]	12	5	7	58			91			72
Philadelphia (95–96) [13]	12	0	12	50			75			67

Ad Adults; *Ch* children

■ Main American single-center series of *ex situ* split

Collectively, there were 64 recipients, comprising 11 adults and 53 children (Tables 4 and 5). These small numbers underline the long lasting reluctance of USA centers to implement this innovative technique. The technique was mostly restricted to high-risk patients; it remained investigational for several years being restricted to pediatric centers with a particular interest in the problem [14]. Overall patient and graft survival rates were similar to the results obtained in Europe, although with a higher incidence of primary non-function.

Table 5. Main American single-center series of *ex situ* split. Percent complications (%)

	n	Bleeding	PNF	Arterial thromb.	Portal thromb.	Biliary	Venous outflow obstruction
Chicago (88–90) [10]	30	22	8	7	8	19	7
Omaha (88–91) [11]	10		17	7	–	20	–
Madison (94–95) [12]	12	–	0	8	–	25	–
Philadelphia (95–96) [13]	12	–	17	–	–	–	–

Table 6. Main series of *in situ* split

	n	Adults	Children	% high risk	Patient survival (%)			Graft survival (%)		
					Ad	Ch	Overall	Ad	Ch	Overall
Hamburg (94–95) [15]	14	7	7	36	100	71	93	86	71	79 (R: 100%)
Los Angeles (96–97) [16]	28	14	12	58	86	100	92	79	92	86

Ad Adults; *Ch* children

In situ split

This technique was pioneered by the Hamburg group [15], followed by the UCLA group [16]. Despite the high proportion of high-risk patients, overall patient and graft survival rates were outstanding, particularly for adult recipients (Tables 6 and 7). The near zero incidence of surgical complications, and particularly of biliary complications, was very remarkable. Of great importance was the 100% functional outcome of other organs retrieved from the same donors.

European split liver transplantation registry

The European experience of *ex situ* split liver transplantation accumulated between 1990–1993 was analyzed by J. de Ville de Goyet [17]. It comprised a total of 87 split grafts (43 right, 44 left); 32 were transplanted in elective patients and 55 in urgent patients.

Table 7. Main series of *in situ* split. Percent complications

	n	Bleeding	PNF	Arterial thromb.	Portal thromb.	Biliary	Venous outflow obstruction
Hamburg (94–95)	14		–	–	–	–	–
Los Angeles (96–97)	28		11	–	–	4	–

100% functional outcome of:	Hamburg	Los Angeles
Kidneys	14	30
Pancreas	2	9
Hearts	5	12
Lungs		7

The overall patient survival rates were 71% for the whole series, 84% for the elective recipients and 65% for the urgent patients without significant differences between recipients of right or left split grafts.

The overall graft survival rates were 62% for the whole series, 73% for the elective recipients and 62% for the urgent recipients, again without significant difference between right and left split grafts. These figures were not different from patient and graft survival rates for full size liver transplants when data were stratified according to the clinical condition of the recipients.

■ European Liver Transplant Registry [18]

Between January 1987 and June 1999, a total of 1036 split grafts (mostly *ex situ*) were transplanted in 898 patients. In adults, the one year patient and graft survival rates were 68% and 60%, respectively. In children (<15 years), the corresponding figures were 75% and 59%, respectively. The survival rates were significantly better in centers having performed more than 40 split transplants.

■ Conclusion

Splitting of the liver graft is a complex surgical procedure. In experienced hands, results are similar to full size liver transplants, although with a higher incidence of biliary complications when the splitting is made *ex situ*. It is not recommended to use this procedure for high-risk patients.

References

1. Pichlmayr R, Ringe B, Gubernatis G, Hauss J, Bunzendahl H (1988) Transplantation of one donor liver to two recipients (splitting transplantation). A new method for further development of segmental liver transplantation. Langenbecks Arch Chir 373:127–130
2. Bismuth H, Morino M, Castaing D, Gillon MC, Descorps Declere A, Saliba F, Samuel D (1989) Emergency orthotopic liver transplantation in two patients using one donor liver. Br J Surg 76:722–724
3. Otte JB, de Ville de Goyet J, Alberti D, Balladur P, de Hemptinne B (1990) The concept and technique of the split liver in clinical transplantation. Surgery 107:605–612
4. Emond JC, Whitington PF, Thistlethwaite JR, Cherqui D, Alonso EA, Woodle IS, Vogelbach P, Busse-Henry SM, Zucker AR, Broelsch E (1990) Transplantation of two patients with one liver. Ann Surg 212:14–22
5. Azoulay D, Astarcioglu I, Bismuth H, Castaing D, Majno P, Adam R, Johann M (1996) Split-liver transplantation. The Paul Brousse Policy. Ann Surg 224:737–748
6. Rela M, Vougas V, Muiesan P, Vilca-Melendez H, Smyrniotis V, Gibbs P, Karani J, Williams R, Heaton N (1998) Split liver transplantation. King's College Hospital Experience. Ann Surg 227:282–288
7. Houssin D, Boillot D, Soubrane O, et al (1993) Controlled liver splitting for transplantation in two recipients: technique, results and perspectives. Br J Surg 80:75–80
8. Mirza DF, Achilleous O, Pirenne J, Buckels AC, McMaster P, Mayer AD (1998) Encouraging results of split-liver transplantation. Br J Surg 85:494–497
9. de Ville de Goyet J (2001) Personal communication
10. Broelsch CE, Emond JC, Whitington PF, Thistlethwaite JR, Baker AL, Lichtor JL (1990) Application of reduced-size liver transplants as split grafts, auxiliary orthotopic grafts, and living related segmental transplants. Ann Surg 212:368–374
11. Langnas AN, Marujo WC, Inagaki M, Stratta RJ, Wood RP, Shaw BW (1992) The results of reduced-size liver transplantation, including split livers, in patients with end-stage liver disease. Transplantation 53:387–391
12. Kalayoglu M, D'Alessandro AM, Knechtle SJ, Hoffmann RM, Pirsch JD, Judd RH, Armbrust M, Spaith E, Pilli G, Young CJ, Geffner SR, Odorico JS, Sollinger HW, Belzer FO (1996) Preliminary experience with split liver transplantation. J Am Coll Surg 182:381–387
13. Dunn SP, Haynes JH, Nicolette LA, Falkenstein K, Pierson A, Billmire DF, Vinocur CD, Weintraub W (1997) Split liver transplantation benefits the recipient of the "leftover liver". J Ped Surg 32:252–255
14. Broelsch CE, Stevens LH, Whitington PF (1991) The use of reduced-size liver transplants in children, including split livers and living related liver transplants. Eur J Pediatr Surg 1:166–171
15. Rogiers X, Malago M, Gawad K, Jauch KW, Olausson M, Knoefel WT, Gundlach M, Bassas A, Fischer L, Sterneck M, Burdelski M, Broelsch E (1996) *In situ* splitting of cadaveric livers. The ultimate expansion of a limited donor pool. Ann Surg 224:331–341

16. Goss JA, Yersiz H, Shackleton C, Seu P, Smith CV, Markowitz JS, Farmer DG, Ghobrial RM, Markmann JF, Arnaout WS, Imagawa DK, Colquhoun SD, Fraiman MH, McDiarmid SV, Busuttil RW (1997) *In situ* splitting of the cadaveric liver for transplantation. Transplantation 64:871–877
17. de Ville de Goyet J (1997) European Split Liver Registry (1990–1993). Transplantation 59:1371–1376
18. European Liver Transplant Registry. Custodian: R. Adam (Villejuif, France)

1.2 Split liver transplantation: what has been done and where is the need

A. Königsrainer, R. Ladurner and R. Margreiter

■ Introduction

Orthotopic full size liver transplantation has become an accepted form of treatment for patients with endstage liver disease and can therefore be considered standard therapy. Survival rates at one and two years reported by the European Liver Transplant Registry (ELTR) are 83% for patients transplanted since 1994. In a few centers results are even better and exceed 90% patient survival at one year. As a consequence of these results indications were broadened, which led to an increase in patients awaiting such a transplant.

If localized primary liver tumors, alcoholic liver disease and the need for liver retransplantation are accepted as indications, the demand for liver transplants can be calculated to be 25 per million population. Since not more than 80% of all donor livers can be used, depending on donor incidence, between 30% and 80% of the demand can be transplanted. Furthermore, only 10% to 20% of the available livers are suitable for splitting [1].

Whereas between December 1997 and December 1998 the number of patients on the Eurotransplant liver waiting list increased by some 30%, the transplantation rate remained the same during the same period. Mortality, and the delisting rate, mainly due to deterioration of a patient's general condition and usually directly associated with poor liver function, was 19%. On the other hand, during this one-year period 7% of the patients received a split graft and 10% of the transplants were performed in children [2].

Strict patient selection is one possible means of preventing death on the waiting list. Considering the natural course of the underlying disease, transplantation still represents the best therapeutic option, even for patients with primary liver tumors. Nor is advanced age considered a contraindication for liver transplantation.

To increase the number of transplants, more and more organs from marginal donors have been accepted in recent years. Transplantation of such organs is associated with a higher morbidity, longer hospital stay and poorer overall outcome; thus, in the case of a marginal donor liver it is crucial that recipients be selected who are fit enough to survive retransplantation, if necessary [3].

ELTR reports a constant retransplantation rate between 10% and 15%, with some centers having a rate of 5% or even less, while at others it is higher than 20%. More than 50% of retransplants are performed during the first month after transplantation and mainly for technical reasons. A recent report seems to demonstrate a strong correlation between transplantation activity and outcome [4].

The rationale for liver splitting is to reduce or prevent mortality on the waiting list, reduce waiting time and prevent deterioration of patient condition. Up to now only in pediatric liver transplantation have new technical alternatives such as the use of reduced-size or segmental grafts as well as living-related transplantation been able to reduce the death rate from about 20% to 0–5% [5]. Even if it must be our goal to increase the number of transplants, splitting a liver must be for the benefit of both recipients and thus for the entire patient population awaiting a transplant.

■ Splitting between child and adult

Size reduction of an adult liver or the use of segments was implemented only to overcome the need for size-matched grafts in pediatric recipients. The remaining liver, however, was discarded and this procedure led to a shift in donor organs from adults to children. Therefore, living-related liver transplantation was introduced as a logical extension of reduced-size and segmental liver transplantation. Both reduced-size and living-related liver transplantation were able to significantly decrease mortality on the waiting list with results equivalent to whole liver transplantation.

As a next step, split liver transplantation was implemented. This technique allows a whole liver to be divided into two allografts and therefore the total number of grafts to be increased. The first clinical case was reported by Pichlmayr et al. in 1988, who gave the right split graft to an adult and the left split graft to a child [6]. Early results, however, were significantly inferior to whole organ transplantation: only 67% of the children and 20% of the adults survived [7]. But results soon improved, as can be seen from the first report of the European split liver registry in 1995, in which the survival rates were stratified according to the recipient status at the time of transplantation. In elective cases patient and graft survival at six months were 89% and 80% for children and 80% and 72% for adults, respectively. When a split graft was transplanted in an urgent situation, patient and graft survival rates were 61% and 61% for infants and 68% and 55% for adults, respectively. Twenty percent of grafts were lost for technical reasons. This retrospective analysis demonstrates that in elective cases split liver transplantation gives results similar to those for whole organ transplantation. The incidence of vascular and biliary complications as well as the primary non-function rate, however, were higher than after whole organ transplantation [8].

The reason is that splitting a liver is a time-consuming procedure usually associated with a longer cold ischemia time and with the risk of some rewarming. Thus, selection of "high-quality organs" and low-risk recipients is mandatory. Furthermore, only a few centers are equipped to allow two recipients to be transplanted at the same time.

A retrospective analysis of survival and morbidity after elective pediatric liver transplantation with full size (FSG) and technical variant grafts (TVG) from a single center was reported by Sieders et al. in 1999 [9]. Of 97 children 47 received an FSG and 50 a TVG. The TVG includes segments and lobes from split and non-split livers. Only hemodynamically stable heart-beating donors with normal or near-normal liver function tests were used. The liver reduction or splitting procedure was done *ex situ* immediately after arrival at the transplant center. The one-, three-, and five-year survival rates for patients after FSG vs TVG were 89% vs 83%, 88% vs 67% and 80% vs 67% and for the graft 77% vs 71%, 77% vs 52%, and 70% vs 52%, respectively. Incidence of biliary, vascular, bleeding, and infectious complications was higher, while the sepsis rate was significantly higher after TVG transplantation. The difference in the overall complication rate and the reintervention rate reached statistical significance ($p < 0.01$). In most instances reintervention and sepsis in TVG were caused by biliary complications.

Splitting the liver *in situ* and carefully transsecting the bile duct for the left lobe or the left lateral segments close to the parenchyma without damaging the vasculature of the right bile duct usually helps prevent biliary complications. It goes without saying that ischemic time should be kept as short as possible.

Based on the experience with living-related liver transplantation the *ex situ* technique was modified as mentioned above and *in situ* splitting developed. In 1997 Rogiers et al. reported their first experience with 14 *in situ* split grafts [10]. The six month patient and graft survival rates were 93% and 85%, respectively. A significantly lower incidence of biliary and bleeding complications as well as a lower initial non-function rate were observed.

How to handle the problem of segment IV during or after the splitting procedure is still a matter of controversy. In order to keep segment IV viable, the artery for segment IV should be preserved whenever possible. It can easily be identified in most heart-beating cadaveric donors. Perfusion of segment IV can be assessed during in vivo dissection. When hypoperfusion is observed in the recipient, atrophy occurs in the majority of cases without creating further complications.

The technique for implanting the right split graft is identical to that for standard orthotopic liver transplantation. Rela et al. reported in 1998 on 19 patients who received a right split lobe. All except one were transplanted for chronic liver disease. After a median follow-up of 12 months one patient had died and no graft losses were observed, giving a patient and graft survival of 95 %. Altogether three biliary complications were seen: two bile leaks from the cut surface were drained percutaneously and one anastomotic stricture had to be treated surgically [11].

According to Eurotransplant allocation rules, pediatric grafts must be given to pediatric recipients. If, however, a child is listed as a high urgent candidate, the first liver available, which in many cases is an adult liver, must be allocated to the child, meaning a size reduction or splitting procedure is usually necessary. More recent results with these procedures seem to justify such an allocation policy.

Living-related liver transplantation has become a valuable alternative to TVG. UNOS data clearly demonstrate the impact of this type of graft on the outcome [12]: live donor graft survival (76%) was comparable with whole liver graft survival (71%), but significantly better at one year than was survival of split liver grafts (60%; $p=0.007$) or reduced-size grafts (61%; $p=0.001$). This holds true even after exclusion of retransplants and ICU-bound recipients. In children less than one year of age, significantly better graft and patient survival rates were achieved with live donor grafts (83% and 89%) than with whole liver grafts (62% and 76%) or reduced-size grafts (63% and 75%). Superior results for living-related liver transplantation would be an argument for extending this option to small and critically ill pediatric patients.

Between 1996 and 1999 a total of 18 children were transplanted at our institution. Six children received a whole liver graft, five a TVG (three split grafts, two reduced-size grafts), and seven a segmental graft from a live donor. One child died one month after a split liver transplantation due to septic complications. All remaining children are currently alive and well. One graft each was lost in the TVG as well as the living-related group due to arterial thrombosis. In one child a bilioma was drained percutaneously after reduced-size transplantation and in another child reoperation was necessary after split liver transplantation for bleeding from the cut surface.

Based on the current literature and our own limited experience we feel that the demand for pediatric liver grafts can be met by using all available pediatric donors and grafts from live donors. Only in cases of highly urgent transplants would it be necessary to use segmental grafts from adult cadaveric donors. It is therefore our policy that the first preference is a whole pediatric liver. Our second option would be a living-related donor, and only if neither of these two options can be realized would a cadaveric segmental graft be chosen.

■ Splitting between adults

There have been few attempts to transplant two adults using a split liver graft. Considering that about 20% of donor livers can be split and used for two adults, the number of transplants could be increased significantly.

To achieve this goal, two major modifications of the current policy are necessary. First, the technique need for the splitting procedure needs to be changed. Splitting the liver in a way that leaves a classical right lobe comprising segments V–VIII and a left lobe consisting of the remaining segments would provide two adult recipients with sufficient liver cell mass. The proposal by Colledan et al. to leave the caval vein with the left lobe will probably solve the technical problems [13]. However, a small patient must be selected for the left hemi-liver since only grafts with more than 1% of the liver volume/recipient body weight ratio or more than 40% of the liver volume are considered sufficient. Transplanting less than 1% can be dangerous and could render an elective patient a highly urgent retransplant candidate.

To keep ischemic injury to a minimum it is crucial that *in situ* splitting be performed whenever possible. Since severe early rejection might suffice to cause failure of a graft with little functional reserve, a more powerful immunosuppression including IL-2 antibodies may be indicated [14].

Thus far, only five splitting procedures for transplantation into ten adults have been reported. Four grafts (three left and one right) failed within weeks of transplantation. Two graft failures were caused by insufficient liver mass [15–17]. Our own experience with four transplants using split grafts into adults was sobering: the recipient of the left lateral segments died and the second patient given segments II–IV had to be retransplanted for insufficient liver cell mass. The calculated volume of segments II and III was 400 ml, corresponding to 0.8% of the liver volume/BW ratio and 582 mL for segments II–IV with a ratio of 1.2%, respectively. Both donors had largely normal liver histology and function.

In order to promote split liver transplantation for adults, changes in organ allocation strategies will be necessary. The left hemi-liver should be allocated to an elective recipient preferably smaller than the donor with a liver/recipient bodyweight ratio greater than 1%. This would make it necessary to create a separate category of potential recipients of a left hemi-liver, i.e., small recipients in good condition. Patients on such a waiting list could espect a shorter waiting time and thus the possibility of being transplanted while still in good general condition. This benefit has to be carefully balanced against the risk of a TVG. It would be only fair enough to thoroughly inform patients of the benefits as well as the risks of such a policy. Implementation of routine liver splitting for two adults on a national basis would be a major step forward and certainly help reduce mortality on the waiting list [14].

In addition, to avoid additional ischemic damage to the left lobe graft it should be transplanted at the donor center, whereas the right lobe would be shipped as usual.

For the sake of completeness it should be mentioned that more and more center, not only in Asia but also in the US and Europe, are adopting programs for live donation of the right liver lobe with excellent results. It must be emphasized, however, that a few donor deaths have already been reported. Therefore, such a procedure must be considered very carefully and carried out only in centers with experience in major hepatic surgery as well as segmental graft liver transplantation.

Conclusion

Splitting a liver for a child and an adult will not solve the current organ shortage. Using pediatric donor livers exclusively for children and promoting live donation together with the possibility of using cadaveric liver segments would eliminate mortality on the pediatric waiting list and benefit the adult patient population. Splitting every splittable organ for two adults using entire right and left lobes could increase the number of grafts by 10%–15%, but requires thoughtful patient selection.

References

1. Busuttil RW, Goss JA (1999) Split liver transplantation. Ann Surg 229:313–320
2. De Meester J (1999) Liver: donation, waiting list, and transplants. In: Eurotransplant International Foundation Annual Report 1988, pp 39–44
3. Malago' M, Rogiers X, Hertl M, Bassas A, Burdelski M, Broelsch CE (1998) Optimization of the use of the cadaveric liver. Transplant Proc 30:3902–3903
4. Edwards EB, Roberts JF, Mc Bride MA, Schulak JA, Hunsicker LG (1999) The effect of the volume of procedures at transplantation centers on mortality after liver transplantation. N Engl J Med 341:2049–2053
5. Otte JB (1995) Is it right to develop living related liver transplantation? Do reduced and split livers not suffice to cover the needs? Transpl Int 8:69–73
6. Pichlmayr R, Ringe B, Gubernatis G, Hauss J, Bunzendahl H (1988) Transplantation einer Spenderleber auf zwei Empfänger (Splitting – Transplantation); eine neue Methode in der Weiterentwicklung der Lebersegment – Transplantation. Langenbecks Arch Chir 373:127–130
7. Broelsch CE, Emond JC, Whitington PF (1990) Application of reduced-size liver transplants or split grafts, auxiliary orthotopic grafts and living related segmental transplants. Ann Surg 214:368–377
8. De Ville de Goyet J (1995) Split liver transplantation in Europe 1988–1993. Transplantation 59:1371–1376
9. Sieders E, Peeters PMJG, Ten Vergert EM, Bijleveld CMA, De Jong KP, Zwaveling JH, Boersma GA, Slooff MJH (1999) Analysis of survival and morbidity after pediatric liver transplantation with full – size and technical – variant grafts. Transplantation 68:540–545
10. Rogiers X, Malago' M, Gawad K, Broelsch CE (1996) *In situ* splitting of cadaveric livers: the ultimate expansion of the donor pool. Ann surg 224:331–341
11. Rela M, Vougas V, Muiesan P, Vilca-Melendez H, Smyrniotis V, Gibbs P, Karani J, Williams R, Heaton N (1998) Split liver transplantation, King's College Hospital experience. Ann Surg 227:282–288

12. Sindhi BR, Rosendale J, Mundy D, Taronto S, Baliga P, Reuben A, Hebra A, Tagge E, Othersen HB (1999) Impact of segmental grafts on pediatric liver transplantation - a review of the United Network for Organ Sharing Scientific Registry Data (1990–1996). J Ped Surg 34:107–111
13. Colledan M, Andorno E, Valente U, Gridelli B (1999) A new splitting technique for liver grafts. Lancet 353:1763 (letter)
14. Strasberg SM, Lowell JA, Howard TK (1999) Reducing the shortage of donor livers: what would it take to reliably split livers for transplantation into two adult recipients? Liver Transplant Surgery 5:437–450
15. Goss JA , Yersiz H, Shackleton CR, Sen P, Smith CV, Markowitz JS (1994) *In situ* splitting of the cadaveric risk factors for poor function after orthotopic liver transplantation. Hepatology 20:829–839
16. Bismuth H, Morino M, Castaing D, Gillon MC, Descorps Declere A, Saliba F, Samuel D (1989) Emergency orthotopic liver transplantation in two patients using one donor liver. Br J Surg 76:722–724
17. Azoulay D, Astarcioglu J, Bismuth H, Castaing D, Majno P, Adam R, Johann M (1996) Split - liver transplantation. The Paul Brousse policy. Ann Surg 224:737–746
18. Kinchi T, Kasahara M, Uryuhara K, Inomata Y, Uemoto S, Asonuma K, Egawa H, Fujita S, Hayashi M, Tanaka K (1999) Impact of graft size mismatching on graft prognosis in liver transplantation from living donors. Transplantation 67:321–327
19. Marcos A (2000) Right lobe living donor liver transplantation: a review. Liver Transplantation 6:3–20

1.3 Logistic aspects and procedures in split liver transplantation

T. KARBE, D.C. BROERING, R. KUETEMEIER, and X. ROGIERS

■ Introduction

The reason for establishing a split liver transplant (SLT) program at the University Hospital of Hamburg was due to the decreasing number of adequate cadaveric donor livers within Eurotransplant and to the increasing necessity of liver transplantations during the same period. As a consequence, the mortality rate of potential recipients on the waiting list, particularly of infants, was increasing, because the number of small-sized donor livers available is small. These circumstances have still not changed. New statistical data show that in 1999 the number of new registrations of patients waiting for a liver transplantation in Germany increased about 6.9% in comparison to 1998. Unfortunately, in the same time period 151 patients died on the waiting list and 70 patients were released because of poor health condition. However, in 1999 757 patients received a liver graft in Germany.

■ The advantages of split liver transplantation

The split liver transplantation gives the opportunity of grafting small children as well as small adults with size-matched organs without reducing the adult cadaveric donor liver pool, that means:

- The transplantation of two patients (normally a small infant and a small adult) by transection in the heart beating donor (*in situ*) or on the backtable (*ex situ*) of one donor liver.
- The transplantation of two small-sized adults by bipertition (full left – full right split) in the heart beating donor (*in situ*) or on the backtable (*ex situ*) of one donor liver.

Before establishing a split liver transplant program some basic requirements should be fulfilled:

- The transplant center should have infants and adults as well as small-sized adults on their waiting list.

The transplant center should have experience in liver surgery techniques, and with reduced-graft transplants.
The transplant center should have sufficient hospital facilities and personnel resources including the availability of two surgical and anesthesiological teams at the same time to run the program.
Cooperation with other transplant centers.

Two aspects for the successful enforcement of an SLT program, which may have a decisive effect on the outcome of transplanted patients, are excellent logistics and coordination. The goal should be to ensure a quick, proper and efficient procedure. Therefore, a smooth proceeding as well as clear structured time schedules are necessary to optimize the complete splitting set-up and to avoid complications.

In fact, the whole logistic machinery should not be activated before having clarified that a splitting procedure is practicable (Fig. 1). For example if there are suboptimum facilities at the donor hospital, the donor liver is better explanted in a "normal fashion" and an *ex situ* splitting should be performed later at the splitting/recipient center. On the recipients' side medical and logistical aspects, like patients' health status and sufficient options of transportation of the recipent and the donor liver to the transplant center, have to be clarified before starting organizational activities.

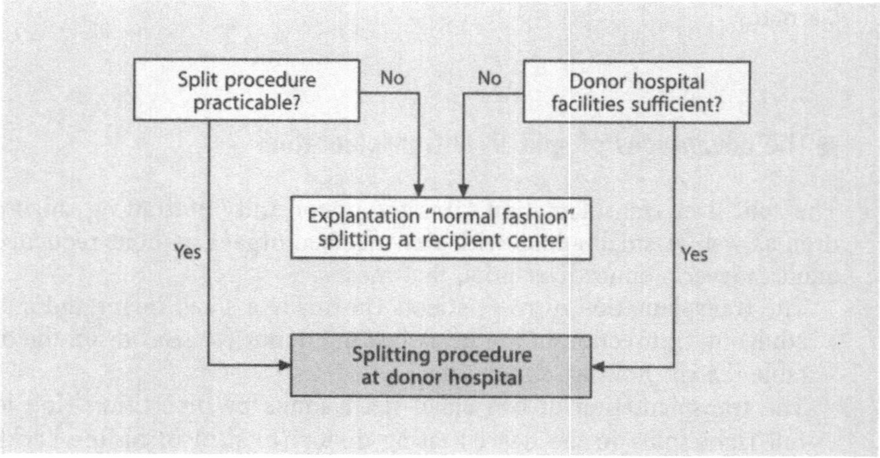

Fig. 1. Principles of coordination in split liver transplantation

■ How does the SLT logistic and coordination work and which activities are necessary in addition to the normal organizational procedure to run a split liver case?

The coordinator is responsible for organization of a split liver transplantation (Fig. 2). First, the coordinator at the splitting/recipient center has to ensure that permission to perform a split liver retrieval has been given by the coordinator of the donor hospital. Next, a suitable time schedule for the liver retrieval at the donor hospital including optimal transport facilities in cooperation with the local coordinator is set. Also, a suitable schedule at the splitting/recipient center has to be arranged, so that OR, ICU, transplant ward and various labs can start organizing their specific logistic contribution. Finally, the Eurotransplant has to be posted regarding the procedure in case of sequential harvesting of both liver halfs.

What different kinds of split techniques are possible.

The *ex situ* splitting: Normal organ procurement, donor liver transection on the backtable after perfusion and liver harvesting (Fig. 3).

The *in situ* split technique: Surgical technique of transection of the donor liver in the heart beating donor, before starting perfusion of the remaining liver and other donor organs. In this case the left lateral segment can be perfused on the backtable.

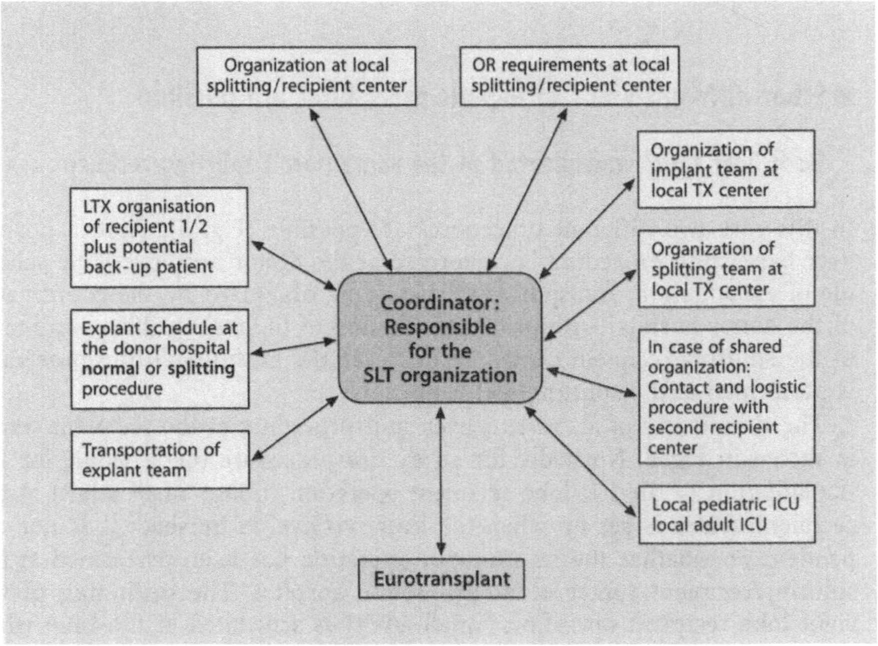

Fig. 2. LTX organization of recipient 1/2 plus potential back up patient

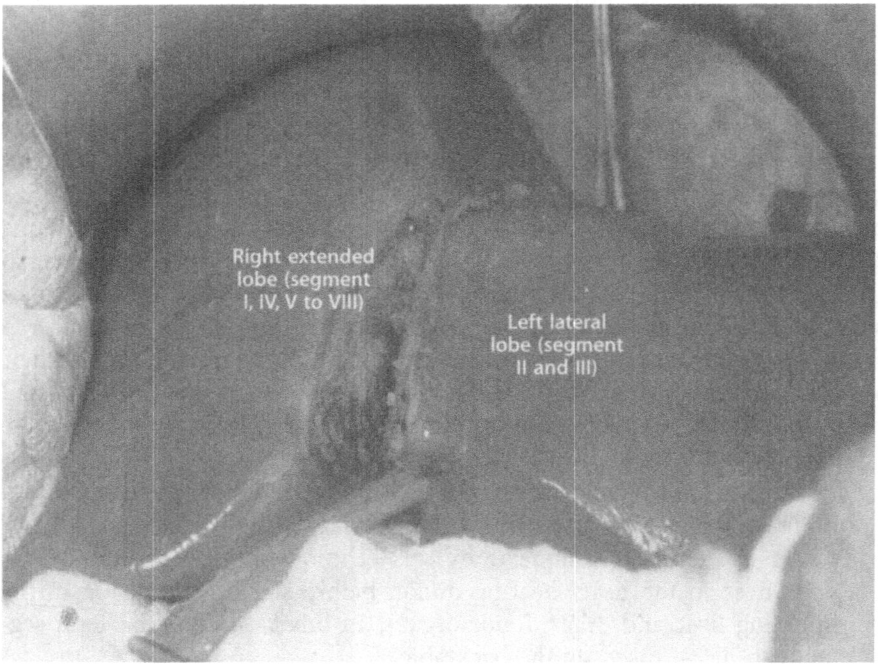

Fig. 3. Left lateral segment after *in situ* splitting

■ What different kinds of logistic procedures are possible

Both liver splits transplanted at the same (local) splitting/recipient center

In this case two different procedures are possible (Fig. 5): First, a normal liver harvesting procedure is performed at the donor hospital. Time schedule of explantation, transport, etc., has to be organized by the coordinator of the donor hospital with prior consultation of the responsible coordinator of the splitting/recipient center. In this case the *ex situ* splitting procedure is performed at the splitting/recipient center.

The time frame of an *ex situ* liver split procedure at the recipient center is shown in Fig. 6. Normally for an *ex situ* procedure the schedule for the implantation of the left lobe recipient operation (infant small adult) at the recipient center is set up when the liver retrieval is finished; it is not dependent on whether the *ex situ* split operation has been performed at the splitting/recipient center or at the donor hospital. The beginning of the right lobe recipient operation (small adult) is scheduled at the time when the reperfusion of the left lobe recipient is completed.

Finally, the surgical team that performed the *ex situ* split begins the implantation of the recipient who is to receive the remaining liver. This allows

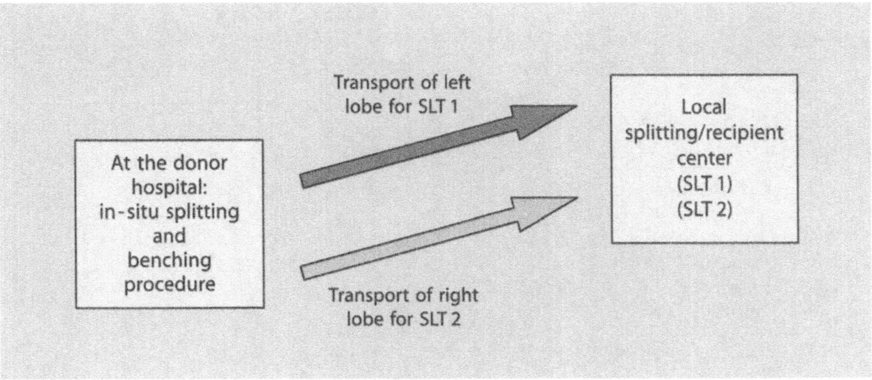

Fig. 4. Split procedure and coordination at the "Local Recipient Center"

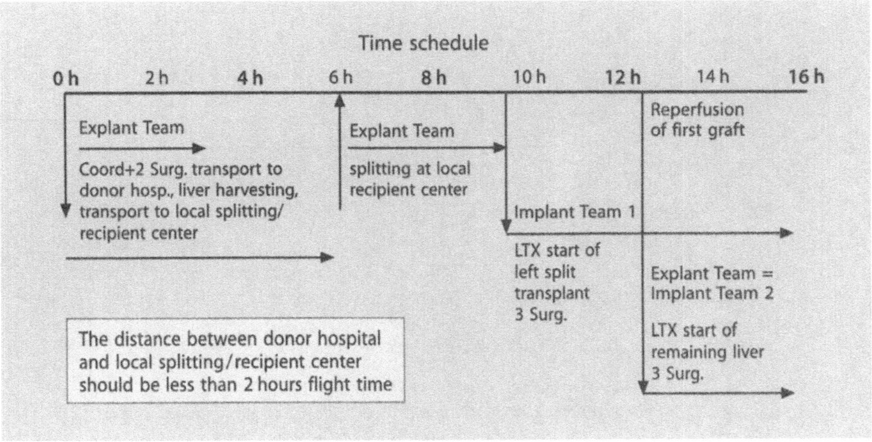

Fig. 5. "EX SITU" split procedure and coordination at the LOCAL splitting/recipient center

the transplantation of both recipients in one transplant center using only two surgical teams and avoids simultaneous reperfusions.

Second, for *an in situ* procedure at the donor hospital, the final decision has to be made very early, namely at the time Eurotransplant offers the donor liver to the splitting/recipient center or when the donor procurement at the donor hospital is in progress in order to start the organization for the recipient's transplantation immediately. In this case, the coordinator of the splitting/recipient center is responsible for the whole logistic in cooperation with the coordinator of the donor hospital (Fig. 7).

However, an optimal time schedule is important for the left lateral liver graft which usually has to be prepared first for implantation (Fig. 8). After flush perfusion and benching of the left segments is completed, one surgeon of the harvesting team has to return to the local splitting/recipient

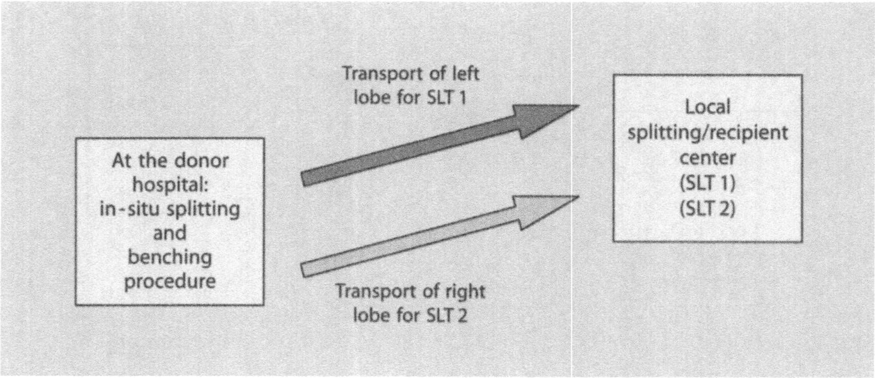

Fig. 6. Split procedure and coordination at the "Local Recipient Center"

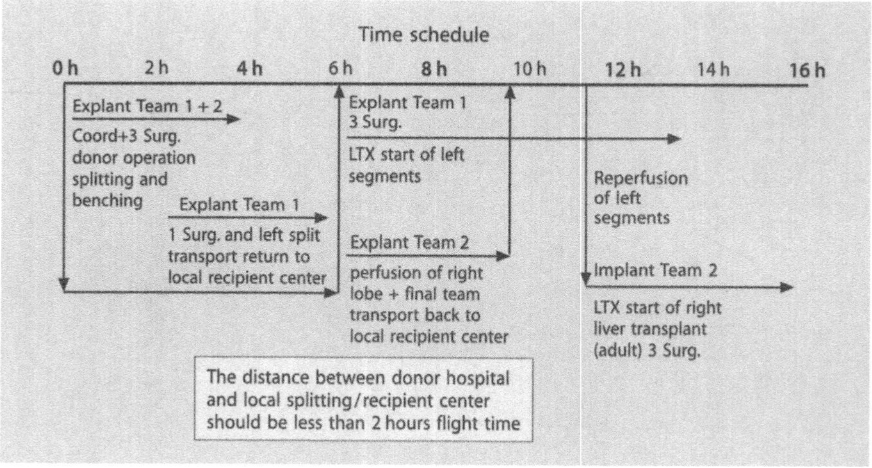

Fig. 7. "IN SITU" split procedure and coordination at the "DONOR HOSPITAL"

center immediately in order to avoid long cold ischemic time. The rest of the explant team harvests the remaining liver by normal procedure. Median time between the explantation of the left segments and the right liver lobe is 90 to 120 minutes. Based on these requirements, in general the transportation time between donor hospital and splitting/recipient center should be less than 2 hours.

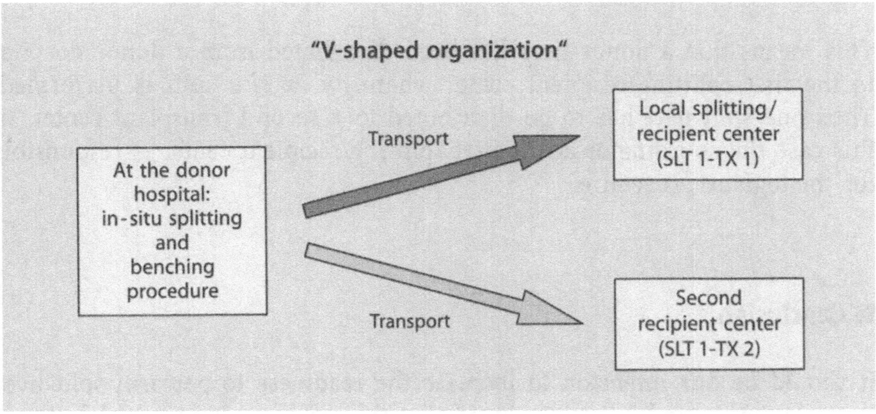

Fig. 8. Shared "IN SITU" split procedure and coordination

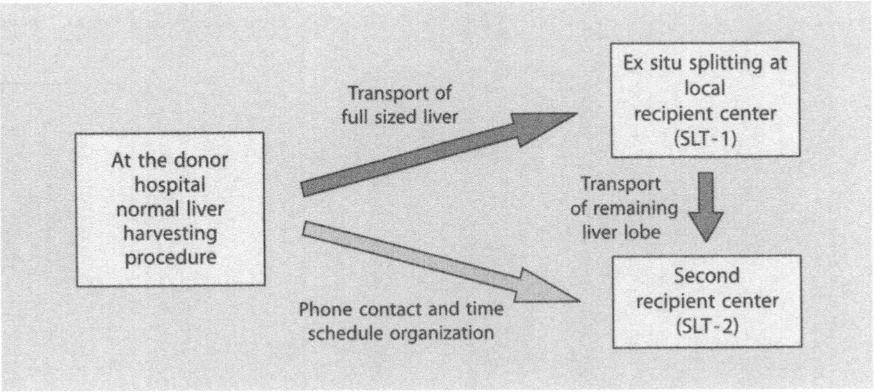

Fig. 9. Shared "TRIANGULAR ORGANIZATION" split procedure and coordination

V-shaped organization procedure

This means that one split (left or right) is grafted at the "local" or first splitting/recipient center and the remaining liver part has to be shuttled to a second transplant center (Fig. 9).

In this case the split procedure (*in situ or ex situ*) always takes place at the donor hospital and the coordinator at the donor hospital is responsible for the transport organization in consultation with the recipient center.

Shared triangular organization procedure

This means that a donor liver has been distributed from a donor hospital to the first splitting/recipient center where *an ex situ* split is performed. Then one split part has to be distributed to a second transplant center. In this case the coordinator at the first splitting/recipient center is responsible for the logistic procedure.

■ Conclusion

It should be our intension to increase the readiness to perform split liver transplantation and I am convinced that this goal can be reached if donor hospitals and transplant centers act in a symbiotic manner because organ donation is a complex task.

1.4 J. Reyes

Allocation policies, logistics, and resource demands of living-related donor and split liver grafts: – the American experience*

■ Background

The growth of segmental graft transplantation has been stimulated by the need to salvage critically ill children awaiting liver transplantation. The first case of reduced liver grafting in a child was performed as an *in situ* procedure in 1972, by Starzl [1]; however, the unsuccessful outcome of this and other sporadic attempts heralded the forthcoming difficulties and controversies of donor surgical technique, recipient selection and implantation, and what to do with the "left-over" liver segment.

Technical advances of liver graft reduction developed by Bismuth [2] in 1983 and Broelsch [3] in 1984 resulted in improvements in patient and graft survival, as well as decrease in pre-transplant mortality. Subsequently in 1989 Dr. Pichlemyer [4] addressed the issue of the "left-over" segment by describing the technique of splitting a liver graft *ex situ* and transplanting two recipients. Nonetheless, the results with such procedures were poor; it was only with technical developments of arterial, biliary, and graft preservation techniques, particularly in the setting of a living donor graft procedure (which essentially utilizes a reduced left lateral segment graft from a living donor), that enhancements in utilization of reduced-size grafts either through living-related donors, reduced liver grafting, or *ex situ* splitting of a cadaveric liver graft was achieved [5]. With the establishment of living-related left lateral segment liver grafting survival comparative to whole organ cadaveric survival, the next step in enhancing graft and patient survival with split liver transplantation came with the introduction of the *in situ* technique by Rogiers [6] in 1985. With this technique, the liver can be split *in situ* (similar to a living-related donor procedure) in the hemodynamically stable cadaveric donor. Consequently, within a period of 10 years the results of split liver transplantation has improved from survival rates of around 50% in 1984 to 90% after 1995 (Table 1).

* Acknowledgment: Supported in part by research grants from the Veterans Administration and Project Grant No. DK-29961 from the National Institutes of Health, Bethesda, MD

Table 1. Published experience with split liver grafts

Center	Year	*In/ex situ*	No.	Patient survival rate %	Graft survival rate %
Emond	1989	*Ex situ*	18	67	60
Thistlewaite	1990	*Ex situ*	28	57	50
Broelsch	1990	*Ex situ*	30	50	43
Shaw	1990	*Ex situ*	10	50	
Otte	1990	*Ex situ*	4	50	50
Slooff	1995	*Ex situ*	15	73	67
Otte	1995	*Ex situ*	29	79	69
De Ville	1995	*Ex situ*	96	71	64
Azoulay	1995	*Ex situ*	27	79	79
Rogiers	1995	Mixed	16	81	75
Rogiers	1996	*In situ*	14	93	86
Kalayoglu	1996	*Ex situ*	12	92	75
Goss	1996	*In situ*	28	92	86
Rela	1998	*Ex situ*	41	90	88
Reyes	2000	*Ex situ*	25	74	61
Reyes	2000	*In situ*	29	96	81

■ American experience: Past and present

National guidelines regarding the utilization of these liver segments has been non-existent. There is no national policy, mandate, or agreement that oversees the utilization of these grafts; nor is there any integration with whole liver allocation activity. At present, living-related donation is a directed donation, and it is generally based on issues regarding preference of the center, ethical questions regarding the specific indications or contraindications, as well as circumstantial factors which would foster, facilitate, or preclude the performance of a living-related donation. Split liver grafting also follows similar guidelines whereby the performance of a split liver transplant is subject to circumstantial factors which would again facilitate this type of graft, such as the ability or preference to perform the procedure as well as the regional opportunity governing the appropriate characteristics of the cadaveric donors. This activity has been performed both on a local basis (usually with an active adult and pediatric program), and through a cooperative effort across regions allowing the sharing of liver segments. In a brief US registry accumulated by Emre [7] and reported at the American Society of Transplant Surgery meeting in 1988, 104 cadaveric liver grafts were split and transplanted into 208 recipients; 62 organs were utilized locally, and 41 organs were shared between centers. In this setting

Table 2. Split liver transplantation (n): the USA experience – centers performing split transplants by year 1988–1996

	1988	1989	1990	1991	1992	1993	1994	1995	1996
1–5	1	3	2	2	3	7	6	7	13
6–10	0	1	0	1	0	0	3	1	3
11–15	1	1	0	0	0	0	0	0	2
16–20	0	0	1	0	0	0	0	0	0
Total	2	5	3	3	3	7	9	8	18

Table 3. Split liver transplantation: the USA experience – split liver transplants by year 1988–1996

1988	1989	1990	1991	1992	1993	1994	1995	1996
16	26	18	12	4	14	32	20	66

of non-existing policies there has been a gradual increase in the number of centers performing split liver transplantation since 1988 when there was a total of 2 centers performing it through 1996 when there were a total of 18 centers performing split liver transplantation (Table 2). The number of procedures done per year has also gradually increased from a total of 16 split liver graftings in 1988 to a total of 66 in 1996 (Table 3).

The pediatric results with segmental transplantation as reported by the UNOS registry in an accumulated experience between 1991 and 1996 shows that during that period of time 2636 whole liver grafts were performed as compared to 246 living-related donations, 89 split graftings, and 438 reduced-liver grafts that were implanted in children. The survival after these various types of transplants were comparable in the whole organ and living donor organ groups; however, they were less satisfactory after split liver and reduced transplants. Close analysis of this data reveals that if the status 1 (very urgent cases) are excluded, the patient and graft survivals are actually quite similar for all types of grafts. This suggests that comparative survival results with different hepatic segmental transplants must take into account not only the technique (living donor, reduced, split *ex vivo/in situ*), but also the clinical status of patients receiving these grafts (Table 4).

The total United States experience [7] between 1988 and 1996 of split liver transplantation included 104 donors producing 208 grafts that were transplanted as follows: shared between 2 children (n=27), shared between child and adult (n=72), shared between 2 adults (n=5). The mortality was 13% (27 patients died), with graft loss of 28% (28 from patient death and 31 after retransplantation), for a retransplantation rate of 15%. There were 11 primary non-functions, 15 hepatic artery thrombosis, and 4 biliary

Table 4. Pediatric liver transplantation: UNOS scientific registry 1991–1996

Kaplan-Meir	Live (246)	Whole (2636)	Split (89)	Reduced (438)
Graft (all)	75.6	70.9	60.3 (0.007)	61.1 (0.001)
Graft (pr.non-ICU)	81.4	8.7	66.6 (0.03)	69.9 (0.012)
Patient (all)	88.4	82.6	82	74.4 (0.001)
Patient (pr.-non-ICU)	92.5	89.9	88.4	88.1

complications reported. The three month graft survival was 68% and the 4 year patient survival was 72%. A similar European experience between 1988 and 1993 reported 50 donors producing 98 grafts that were transplanted with a mortality of 27%, graft loss of 36%, and a retransplantation rate of 18%, again mainly due to issues of primary non-function, hepatic artery thrombis, and biliary complications.

The survival analysis of the different American published series reveal that over time and the inevitable learning curves accrued with any novel technique, the *in situ* and *ex situ* techniques are comparably effective and should be performed based on preference and ability since they have equivalent results (Table 1). Similar results from the European experience reported by de Ville de Goyet [8] in 1995, as well as the Pittsburgh experience [9] substantiate similar survivals for the *ex situ* and *in situ* technique.

Transplantation logistics with both *in situ* versus *ex situ* techniques hinge on decrease in cold ischemia times. With the *in situ* technique, since the liver is split at the time of organ procurement the liver can be sent to both hospitals simultaneously, thus, decreasing the ischemia time. This has been further elaborated by Rogiers [6] and others where bringing down cold ischemia times to approximately 12 hours, transplantation graft survival using whole, living-related, and split techniques were similar.

The ideal donor for this type of cadaveric donation is generally between the ages of 15 to 45 and hemodynamically stable. Exclusionary criteria have included malignancy, sepsis, greater than 2 vasopressors, history of hepatitis, a situation which would give a greater than 12 hours cold ischemia time, or cardiac arrest time of greater than 30 minutes, obesity, and alcohol abuse. The results with these techniques will depend also on the selection of the recipients. Most centers feel that any child is a satisfactory recipient; however, high-risk adult patients should be avoided [9]. Consequently the progress with split liver transplantation will hinge on the appropriate selection of donors, recipients, and the appropriate conditions in which the recipients are transplanted.

Such selection of optimal donors also identifies adequate anatomy for division of the organ, and would also point out the situations were we would need to avoid transplantation in the higher risk or technically difficult recipients. Improvements in techniques regarding biliary and vascular reconstructions have also improved the results with splitting. These technical refinements also reflect the learning curve that will need to be achieved by the various centers, hopefully with the assistance of the centers that are already performing these types of split liver grafts. Whether or not these procedures are performed *in situ* or *ex situ*, and the circumstances of the sharing is key to the development of this procedure. Consequently, the transplantation logistics are worked out between the two centers, trying to avoid prolonged ischemia times. Operating room time can be limited to 3 hours, or as little as 1 hour depending on the type of technique utilized. The two sharing surgical teams can resolve the issues of *ex situ* versus *in situ* technique, together with the appropriate placement of the organs. Blood requirements are minimal and should not be a determinant of the feasibility of this procedure. Resource/utilization issues have involved mainly prolongation of operating room time and equipment, and the utilization of blood. However, most organ procurement organizations are actually able to bill for two organs which would eventually decrease procurement costs to the patient and the center.

■ The national split liver policy

The split liver graft allocation policy which establishes a national sharing arrangement for these grafts was proposed and accepted in June 1999 (Table 5). It establishes the donor criteria, and makes recommendations regarding the allocation process for the split liver graft. It is a voluntary participation with the limitation of technique determined by the local preference as far as the left over segment of the split graft, the local center has the right of first refusal of the split liver graft, and it was recommended that affiliation of a pediatric only program with an adult program be a preference in order to enhance the utilization of these segments. There would be an annual review for compliance with this participation.

Table 5. National split liver graft (SLG) policy

- National Sharing arrangement for SLG (June 1999)
- Establishes donor criteria
- Establishes allocation process for SLG
  - Voluntary participation
  - Technique determined by local preference
  - Right of first refusal of SLG belongs to donor program (UNOS Policy 3.6)
  - Affiliation of pediatric only programs with an adult program of preference
- Semi-annual review for compliance
- **Result:** Inclusion in National Liver WLG allocation

Table 6. Split liver transplantation: donors (UNOS) annual report – 1997)

Year	Listed	Death	Donors 6–10	Donors 11–49
1988	566	64	107	1416
1989	587	40	121	1827
1990	629	63	124	2202
1991	666	52	130	2356
1992	763	68	130	2396
1993	826	88	133	2629
1994	891	96	143	2866
1995	820	81	158	2910
1996	859	78	140	2856

However, this type of allocation policy would allocate livers according to the national liver whole organ allocation plans. It is evident from UNOS registry data and its annual report in 1997 that there is a growing demand for pediatric segments with a growing list of children awaiting transplantation from 556 in 1988 to 859 in 1996 (Table 6). Though the number of deaths remain stable, at about 70 to 80 children per year which represents a lower percentage of the total number of patients waiting, it is a persistent mortality. During similar time periods analyzing potentially splitable organs in donors between the ages of 11 and 49, there were well over 1000 donors per year, and in 1996, 2,856 donors met this criteria. Thus, the potential for this resource of split liver grafting is extensive. Further, UNOS registry data between 1990 and 1996 reveals that there is a growing number of pediatric donors available for transplantation; however, with a gradual decrease in the number of pediatric donor organs actually used in pediatric recipients [10].

There are 105 pediatric liver transplant centers in the United States at the present time, and potentially all could have the resources in terms of donors, as well as the need in terms of pediatric recipients. Participation of all of these centers in the national split policy would be ideal. The allocation of the segments follows regional distribution which governs whole organ liver grafting activity. Unfortunately, this limited participation inevitably will restrict the growth and simultaneous progress along a national learning curve. This broader learning curve has been seen, shared, and optimized with the European sharing agreement for split liver grafts across national boundaries. Similarly there is no allocation policy for living-related donor, but more so there is no policy in the event of a failure of a living-related donor graft. Such lack of policy in no way protects the recipient of the living-related donor in the event of post-transplant failure. There is also no incentive for living-related donation since there is no compensation or ability to foster preferred status for living-related donor recipients who have failed. This inevitably is a result of the lack of integration with the whole liver allocation activity.

■ Strategies for increasing split liver transplantation

In any generation of policy for living-related donor and split liver grafts it is important to strive towards a goal of universal interest. Specifically for the donor this would mean screening every potential cadaveric donor that meets limited criteria for split liver grafting. Stop wastage of potentially splitable organs by banning reduced-size grafts as being presently done. Develop both *ex situ* and *in situ* expertise widely among all centers, particularly pediatric centers, and wider sharing of the left-over segment. For the recipients shared goals would mean zero or minimization of waiting times for the critically ill recipients. Minimization of pre-transplant mortality, and maximizing post-transplant outcomes with appropriate selection of splitable organs and appropriate selection of recipients, who would receive these splits. It would also provide incentives to living-related donation in order to optimize this source of donors. Shared goals for a national learning curve would mean the development of technical and administrative advances to broaden application of split liver grafting, for example, as in adult to adult splits, and eventually also auxiliary transplantation, particularly for fulminant hepatic failure and/or failed transplants, and/or inborn errors of metabolism. There should be rigorous follow-up data analysis and communication to participants in any national policy to enhance the development of this learning curve. There should be incentives for the participating centers.

This would translate into the development of a living-related donor and a split liver graft registry. This would be prospective versus retrospective data registry to compare trends and outcomes. It would follow the utilization trends, thus, optimizing this utilization for donor and type of recipient in a prospective analysis form. It would also focus on evolving the standards for split liver graft allocation guidelines and sharing, and it would integrate regional, superregional, national and international experience towards a cooperative effort. Such a registry would provide a periodic real time interactive forum to discuss problems, contemporary issues and controversies. It would provide periodic updates of existing experience in an interactive web site and at national meetings.

Such an interactive web site could also be utilized ideally for the communication of need (real time and the registration of need) real time. Such a registry and interactive registration site for communication of a need in real time response to such need would eventually translate into providing timely transplantation for life saving intent. But without providing incentives for sharing split liver grafts for life saving intent such outcomes would be impossible. Therefore, such incentives could perhaps mean for the donor (living-related donor) high priority to living-related recipients with primary non-function or graft failure from hepatic artery thrombosis. For the recipient of living-related donor/split liver grafts high priority in the event of primary non-function. For the organ procurement organization this would translate into double reimbursement, and should also be viewed as a benchmark for performance from most organ procurement organizations in terms of their ability to refer and to accomplish split liver transplantation. For transplant centers the ability to have left-over segments widely shared could eventually translate into the development of a feasible payback mechanism that would focus on potentially transplanting according to need and for life saving intent, and the transplant center would not lose their segment because there would be a payback system. For transplant personnel there is always the appropriate reimbursement for the development of this new expertise and enhanced activity.

We conclude then that living-related donation and split liver grafting should be based on a need-based sharing for life saving intent ideally on a web site interactive registration site for split liver grafts (*www.needsplit.org*).

■ References

1. Starzl TE, Demetris AJ (1990) Development of the replacement operation. In: Shorpenning NE (ed) Liver Transplantation: A Current Problems in Surgery Classic. Chicago, IL, Year Book Medical Publishers, pp 3–42
2. Bismuth H, Houssin D (1984) Reduced-sized orthotopic liver graft in hepatic transplantation in children. Surgery 95:367–370
3. Broelsch CE, Neuhaus P, Burdelski M et al (1984) Orthotopic transplantation of hepatic segments in infants with biliary atresia. Langenbeck Archiv Chir Forum (Suppl):105–109
4. Pichlmayr R, Ringe B, Guberantis G et al (1989) Transplantation einer Spenderleber auf Zwei Empfänger (Split liver transplantation) Eine neue Methode in der Weitzentwicklung der Lebesegment Transplantation. Lagenbecks Archiv Chir 373:127–130
5. Broelsch CE, Emond JC, Whitington PF et al (1990) Application of reduced-size liver transplants as split grafts, auxillary orthotopic grafts and living-related segmental transplants. Ann Surg 214:368
6. Rogiers X, Malago M, Habib N et al (1995) *In-situ* splitting of the liver in the heart-beating cadaveric organ donor for transplantation in two recipients. Transplantation 59:1081–1083
7. Emre S (1998) American Society of Transplant Surgery Meeting, Chicago
8. Ville De Goyet J (1995) Split liver transplantation in Europe – 1988 to 1993. Transplantation 59:1371–1376
9. Reyes J, Gerber D, Mazariegos GV et al (2000) Split-liver transplantation: A comparison of ex-vivo and *in situ* techniques. J Pediatr Surg 35(2):283–290
10. Sindhi R, Rosendale J, Mundy D et al (1999) Impact of segmental grafts on pediatric liver transplantation – a review of the United Network for Organ Sharing Scientific Registry Data (1990–1996). J Pediatr Surg 34:107–111

2 Anatomy

2.1 G. Kazemier and J.F. Lange

Anatomy of the liver

"La race humaine veut des ideés simples.
Or, le réel est compliqué"
C. Couinaud

Thorough knowledge of anatomy and anatomical variations are prerequisites for liver transplantation. In whole organ liver transplantation, knowledge of anatomy of hilar structures and hepatic veins is necessary but in split liver transplantation additional insight in intrahepatic anatomy is of paramount importance to ensure two viable grafts of sufficient size and with usable vascular and biliary tributaries. Understanding of the concept of functional anatomy and segmentation of the liver represents the basis for splitting the liver for transplantation purposes. In this chapter both the concept of functional anatomy of the liver and the descriptive anatomy of the hepatoduodenal ligament, the intraparenchymal branches of the portal triads and hepatic veins are pointed out. Both aspects are covered with splitting the liver for transplantation in mind. However, the next chapter focuses entirely on the consequences of liver anatomy for the splitting surgeon.

■ Morphological anatomy

The liver is divided by the falciform ligament and the dorsal umbilical fissure into a right and a left lobe. The dorsal intraperitoneal surface of the liver is located in an oblique plane, 45° to the frontal plane. On the visceral aspect of the right lobe the gallbladder fossa, the transverse hilar fissure and the umbilical fissure demarcate the quadrate lobe on the lateral, posterior and medial side, respectively.

The liver is suspended by
the inferior vena cava,
the lesser omentum,
the hepatoduodenal ligament,

the falciform and round ligaments and
the two coronary ligaments, stretching transversely and constituting the right and left triangular ligaments.

The liver surrounds the inferior vena cava; medially the caudate lobe and laterally the posterior parts of the right liver lobe are in close relation to it. The inferior vena cava ligament connects these two, running posteriorly to the inferior vena cava. Suprahepatically on its anterior side the inferior vena cava receives the three larger hepatic veins. The caudate lobe and to a lesser extend the posterior parts of the right lobe drain directly into the inferior vena cava. The lesser omentum with its insertion between the left lobe and the caudate lobe covers the latter on the anterior side and must be divided to expose the common hepatic artery. On the lateral side of the lesser omentum, the hepatoduodenal ligament is encountered, and usually contains the proper hepatic artery, the common bile duct and the portal vein. The two peritoneal layers of the falciform and round ligaments define the medial border of the left lobe of the liver. The round ligament represents the mostly obliterated umbilical vein and it runs from the umbilicus to the portal sinus in the left liver lobe. During the embryological phase, this portal sinus or Rex' sinus is connected to the left hepatic vein and the inferior vena cava by the venous duct of Arantius. The latter obliterates to form the venous ligament and it persists as a fibrous band on the anterior side of the caudate lobe defining the posterior border of the left lobe. Cranially the two coronary ligaments attach the liver to the diaphragm. They are connected to the fibrous sheath of Glisson which encapsulates the entire liver except for the 'bare area' between the left and right coronary ligaments. This Glisson's capsule fuses at the hilum with the connective tissue sheaths surrounding the biliary and vascular structures forming the hilar plate. These connective tissue sheaths surround the portal triads in the liver parenchyma.

■ Functional anatomy and segmentation of the liver

Besides from the four lobe morphological appearance of the liver with its small left lobe, its greater right lobe divided by the falciform ligament and umbilical fissure, its quadrate and caudate lobes a functional anatomy can be discerned. The history of this functional liver anatomy which is clearly described by Strasberg [1] begins with James Cantlie in 1897 who studied liver anatomy by injection of ink into the portal vein [2]. He showed that the line from the fundus of the gall bladder to the inferior vena cava divides the liver into a left and right half, or "true lobes" as he called it. This concept was further developed by McIndoe and Counseler in 1924 using casts of the portal vein, hepatic artery, and bile ducts [3]. In 1948 Hjortsjö published a paper describing examinations of corrosion casts combined with radiographs of the lead enhanced cast material depicting secondary divisions of the liver especially of the ductal system on the right side [4]. In 1953 Healey and Schroy used the same method to show second and third divisions of the ductal system [5]. They recognized segments draining into secondary biliary branches and they used the biliary system as the main guide to describe hepatic divisions.

In 1957 Couinaud published his now classical study on hepatic anatomy [6]. His division of the liver is based upon the distribution of portal veins and the location of the hepatic veins in the parenchyma. In his perception the three hepatic and four portal vein branches are interdigitating fingers dividing the liver into four sectors each receiving one portal pedicle. The four sectors divided by the three hepatic veins are called *portal sectors*, the scissures containing the hepatic veins are called *portal scissures* or *portal fissures*. The scissures containing portal pedicles are called *hepatic scissures*. Couinaud describes the tertiary division of the liver as segments. He recognized eight of these segments which he numbered I–VIII, beginning with the caudate lobe as segment I (Fig. 1). In this chapter and throughout this book the functional division of the liver as advocated by Couinaud is used to describe the different resection planes because this portal segmentation is least prone to anatomical variants [7].

According to the functional anatomy the liver is divided into two hemilivers by the main portal scissure. The right hemiliver is divided by the right portal scissure or tract of the right hepatic vein into an anterior (segments V and VIII) and a posterior sector (segments VI and VII). Care should be taken with regard to segments VI and VII as they are located posteriorly rather than laterally as often described. This mistake is easily understandable as many anatomists were traditionally studying cadaveric livers spread out on a table thus rotating the posterior segments to the lateral side. The left hemiliver is divided by the left portal scissure or tract of the left hepatic vein into an anterior (segments IV and III) and a posterior (segment II) sector. The portal sinus of Rex in the umbilical fissure divides the anterior sector into segments IV and III. Segment I or the caudate lobe can receive its vessels from both left and right portal vein and hepatic artery, and it drains directly into the vena cava and is thus somewhat autonomous as compared to the other segments.

The total liver volume has a relation to body weight and body surface area (2–2.7% of body weight) and in general, the left hemiliver comprises one-third of the total liver volume in adults [8, 9]. However, the ratios between left and right liver volumes may vary considerably between individuals [9]. This makes it unpredictable preoperatively to determine whether splitting the liver will provide adequate grafts for both recipients. Intraoperative or preoperative imaging can be an essential part of the donor work-up particularly when splitting a cadaveric donor for two adult recipients or during living donor liver transplantations [9].

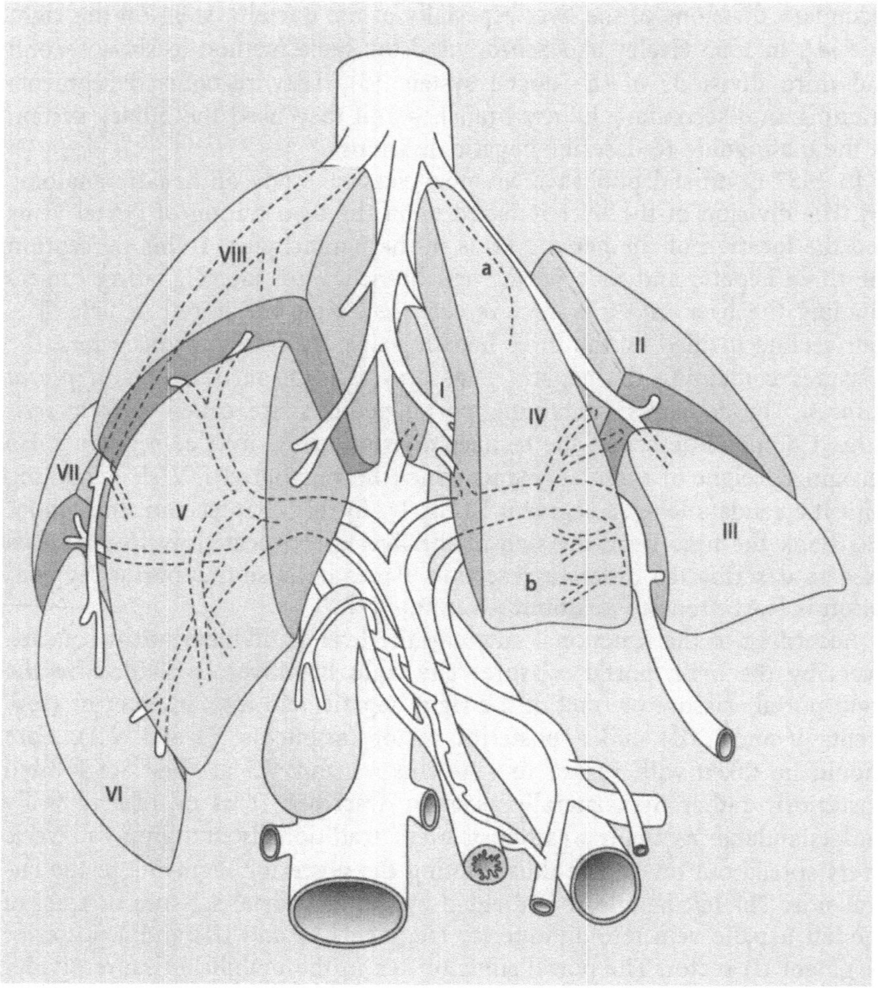

Fig. 1. Segmental anatomy of the liver according to Couinaud

■ Anatomy of the hepatoduodenal ligament and liver hilum

The right lateral margin of the lesser omentum or gastrohepatic ligament contains the proper hepatic artery ventromedially, the portal vein dorsally and the common bile duct in the middle laterally (Fig. 1).

Arterial anatomy

The liver receives blood from two sources: the hepatic artery and the portal vein. The hepatic artery and portal vein provide about 25% and 75% of blood flow, respectively, and both provide 50% of the oxygen. In its regular pattern (75% of cases), the common hepatic artery originates from the celiac trunk and divides into the gastroduodenal and proper hepatic arteries and subsequently into a left and right hepatic artery [10]. Aberrant hepatic arteries are referred to as *accessory* when they occur in addition to the normal arterial supply or as *replaced* when they represent the primary supply to the (hemi) liver. Several authors have described aberrant arterial anatomy but basically, these variants can be summarized as follows: 1) an aberrant common hepatic artery from the superior mesenteric artery; 2) an aberrant left hepatic artery from the left gastric artery; 3) an aberrant right hepatic artery from the superior mesenteric artery [11]. These aberrant arteries can either be replaced or accessory.

In the presence of a hepatic artery bifurcating into a right and left hepatic artery, this bifurcation is typically located close to the division into the gastroduodenal and proper hepatic arteries. Consequently the extrahepatic course of the left and right hepatic artery is long. In most cases the right hepatic artery crosses posteriorly to the common hepatic duct to the lateral side and the right hemiliver. However, it sometimes crosses the bile duct anteriorly. The left and in some cases middle hepatic arteries (supplying segment IV) run on the left side of the bile duct anteriorly to the portal vein. The middle hepatic artery originates in most cases from the left hepatic artery but can also originate from the right hepatic artery (especially in the presence of a replaced left hepatic artery from the left gastric artery) or both or directly from the proper hepatic artery [7]. If it runs extrahepatically it usually crosses the left hepatic duct and left portal vein anteriorly, supplying segment IV. The left hepatic artery usually runs along with the left hepatic duct to supply segments II and III.

The course of the cystic artery has many variations. The typical course is a single cystic artery from the right hepatic artery; however a cystic artery originating from the left or proper hepatic artery and running anteriorly to the bile duct can cause difficulties of interpretation. However, no variant will result in the inability to split a liver for transplantation purposes.

Portal vein anatomy

The portal vein receives blood mainly from the superior mesenteric and splenic veins. Its course in the hepatoduodenal ligament is without variation in most cases. At the liver hilum, the portal vein divides into two veins in 85% of cases; however, in 15% a trifurcation is present [6]. In the case that no right portal vein exists but a trifurcation is present, the branches to the right half of the liver are always right posterior sectorial branches to segments VI and VII and anterior sectorial branches to segments V and VIII, respectively [6, 7, 12]. The course of the left portal vein is relatively long and easily accessible to surgery as it is covered only by peritoneum or a small bridge of liver parenchyma. At the hilum, portal branches to segment I may arise extrahepatically from the left portal vein or the right or from both [6].

Bile duct anatomy

The bile duct at the hepatoduodenal ligament and liver hilum normally follows an extrahepatic course from its confluence very similar to that of the portal vein. The confluence is located at a more cranial level than the portal vein or hepatic artery bifurcation. The cystic duct can drain into the common hepatic duct at various levels. Several variations of ectopic drainage of intrahepatic ducts into the gallbladder and cystic duct, all of which are only rarely of clinical significance during split liver transplantation, have been described [13]. Of greater relevance are the variations of the biliary confluence in the hepatic hilum (Fig. 2a) [5, 6, 14]. Particularly variants with drainage of the branches of the right hemiliver into the left hepatic duct should be noted at cholangiography as these variants can easily result in damage to that left duct during splitting. Intraoperative cholangiography seems essential to tackle these anatomical variations in ductal anatomy during splitting.

The arterial blood supply to the bile duct is of utmost importance during split liver transplantation. Arterial blood supply to the extrahepatic bile duct was described extensively in 1979 by Northover and Terblanche [15]. According to them the blood supply of the supraduodenal duct arises from the retroduodenal, the gastroduodenal, the cystic and the right hepatic arteries and is essentially axial [15]. The most important vessels run on the lateral side of the hepatic duct (Fig. 1). The intrahepatic and the left and right bile ducts are surrounded by a vascular plexus which is derived from branches of the left and right hepatic artery and the segmental branches [16]. This plexus around the intrahepatic ducts is considered an important connection between the hepatic arteries and the gastroduodenal artery via the common duct arteries on the lateral and medial side of the common bile duct. The authors postulate that the caudate lobe, by virtue of its bilateral portal and arterial supply in most cases, represents an important bridge for collateral flow between the left and right hemiliver. One should be aware that, after splitting of the liver through the main portal fissure, these possible collaterals are non-functional. It is suggested to cut the duct back fairly close to the parenchymal cut surface as to provide optimal arterial blood supply to the ductal stump and future anastomotic site.

■ Intrahepatic anatomy

Most of the intraparenchymal anatomy is described in the next chapter dealing with consequences of the liver anatomy for the splitting surgeon. Many of the variants of the main biliary confluence, which are described

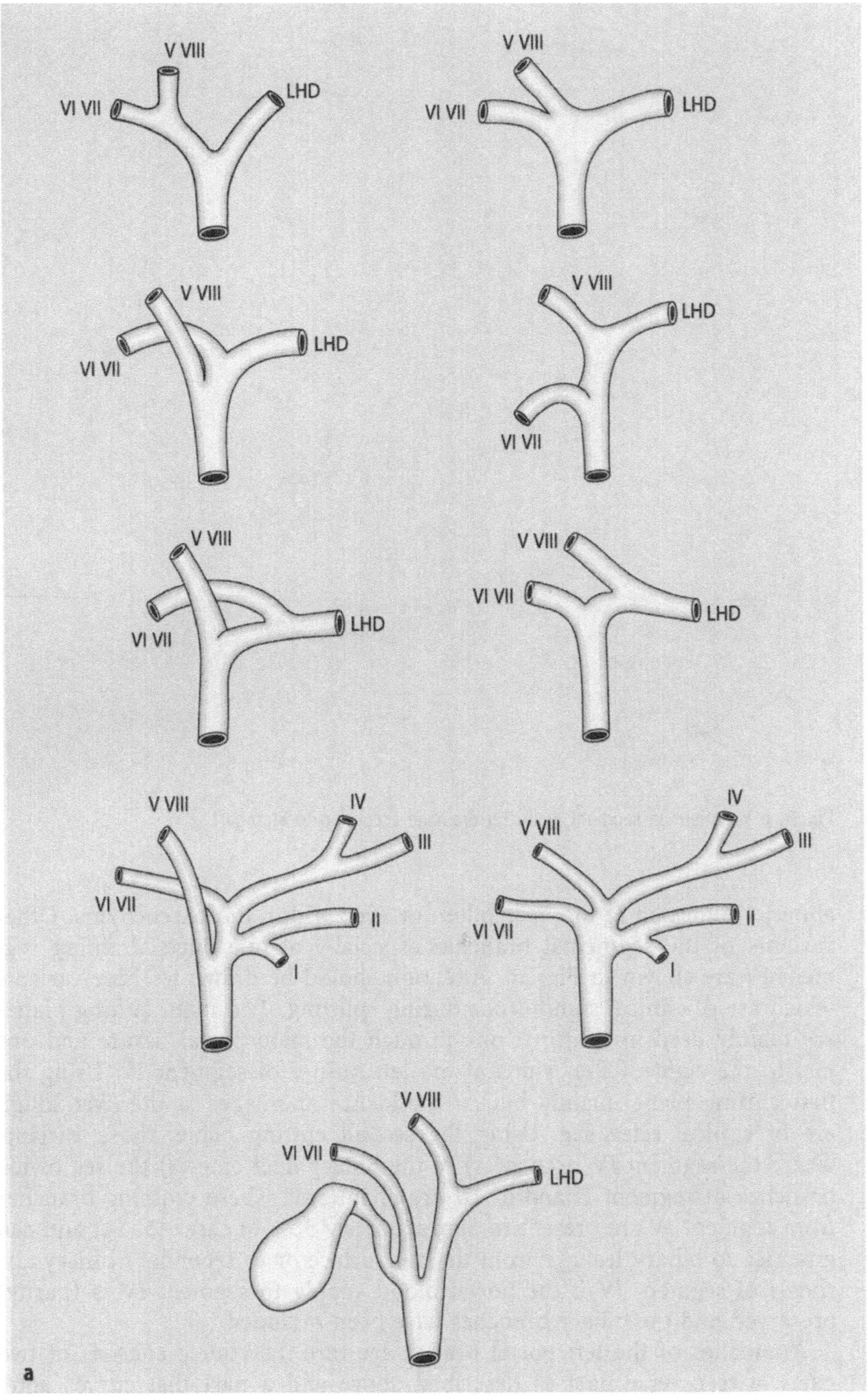

Fig. 2. a Variations in biliary confluence anatomy according to Blumgart

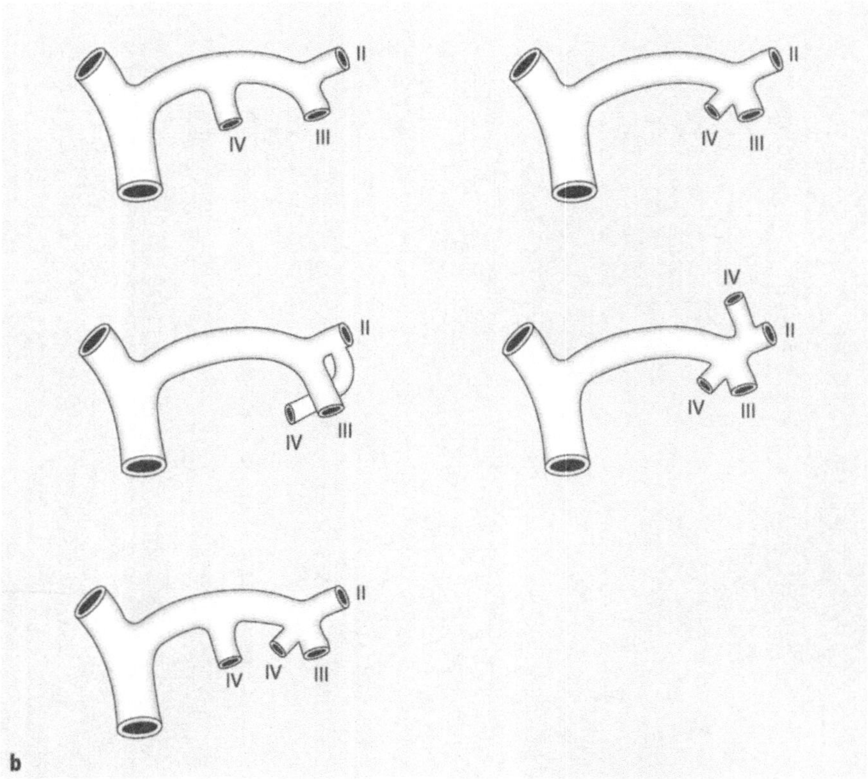

Fig. 2. b Variations in segment IV ductal drainage according to Blumgart

above, are located at the liver hilum or even within the parenchyma. Other variants of the segmental branches especially of bile ducts draining segment IV are shown in Fig. 2b. Attention should be drawn to these variants which are of clinical significance during splitting. Two main cutting planes are mainly used in splitting: one through the main portal fissure and one just to the right of Rex' sinus at the left border of segment IV. Using the first cutting plane, mainly biliary confluence anomalies at the liver hilum are of clinical relevance. Using the second cutting plane, those variants where the segment IV branch(es) of the biliary duct enter(s) the segmental branches of segment II and/or III are of interest. These crossing branches from segment IV are present in approximately 30% of cases [5, 14] and can give rise to biliary leakage from the cut surface or to secondary biliary cirrhosis of segment IV if the portal blood supply to segment IV is (partly) preserved and the biliary branches have been occluded.

Anomalies of the left portal branch are rare. Its course consists of two parts: a transverse part as described above and a part that curves anteriorly, ending at the round ligament, the sinus of Rex. From this sinus, branches to segments II, III and IV originate. The vein to segment II is nearly always solitary [17]. Portal blood flow to segment III is from one (30% of cases), two (38% of cases), or three veins (22% of cases) [17]. From the right part of Rex' sinus, 6–9 portal branches are present supplying segment IV [16]. However, 2–3 portal branches can arise from the transverse left portal vein also supplying segment IV.

The right portal vein is more subject to anomalies than the left [17]. In 15–20% of cases it may not exist, either because

a trifurcation is present, as described above,

the posterior sectorial branches arise directly from the main portal vein and the anterior sectorial branches from the left portal vein or

the posterior sectorial branch divides earlier from the main portal trunk [17].

Many of the variants of the *segmental* portal branches in the right hemiliver are of no clinical relevance to the splitting surgeon as no cutting plane right to the main portal fissure is frequently used.

The arterial bifurcation is always located extrahepatically and therefore most of the anomalies are easily seen during dissection of the hepatoduodenal ligament or the hepatic hilum. Most of the arterial branch anomalies consist of segment IV arterial branches or middle hepatic artery branches. These aberrances are described above. One should be aware that many of the variants are accessory rather than replaced arteries which means that other arterial branches supply the particular segment or sector as well or that collateral circulation exists with those arterial branches [11].

■ Anatomy of the hepatic veins

The venous drainage of the liver into the inferior vena cava typically consists of two major veins: the right hepatic vein, draining mainly the right hemiliver and a common trunk, draining mainly the left hemiliver (Fig. 3). This common trunk arises from the confluence of the left and middle hepatic veins. The right and left inferior diaphragmatic veins typically enter on the right and left side into the right hepatic vein and common trunk, respectively. This confluence is located very cranial in these veins, sometimes joining the suprahepatic inferior vena cava directly.

By definition the right, middle and left hepatic veins run in the right, main and left portal fissure. The right hepatic vein is easily controlled extrahepatically and normally it consists of a trunk without branches prior to its confluence with the vena cava [18]. Control of the left and middle vein separately extrahepatically is less easy in most cases as the confluence of the middle and left hepatic veins into the common trunk is located intrahepatically.

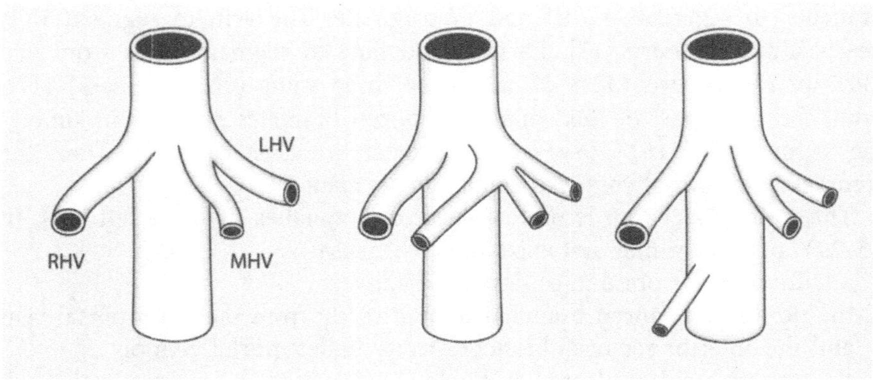

Fig. 3. Main variations in hepatic vein anatomy

The pattern of drainage of different areas of the liver is prone to variation. In addition one should be aware that portal veins usually substitute as draining veins as venous blood flow becomes congested [11, 19]. If this phenomena occurs, no congestion will be noted but portal blood flow towards that area of the liver might be considerably diminished.

The right hepatic vein drains the posterior segments VI and VII, parts of segment VIII and parts of segment V. The middle hepatic vein drains large portions of segments V and VIII and the major part of segment IV. The left hepatic vein drains segments II and III, and a small portion of segment IV [20].

In addition to these three veins, numerous veins, from segments I, VI and to a lesser extent VII drain directly into the vena cava. Drainage of segment I consists mainly of one or two dominant veins and several smaller ones. Apart from the smaller veins from the posterior sector of the right lobe draining directly into the vena cava, in 20–25% of cases one or more short veins, called inferior hepatic veins or Makuuchi veins, drain large portions of segments VI and/or segment VII [11, 20]. Two branches draining anterior parts of the left lateral segment and parts of segment VIII, respectively, might enter very close to the orifice of the left and right hepatic veins or even directly into the vena cava [11, 18].

■ Conclusion

Splitting the liver for transplantation purposes or living donor transplantation challenges the liver surgeon's skills and anatomical expertise. Thorough knowledge of the hepatic anatomy will enable him to overcome almost all variants. If possible preoperative imaging by CT, MRI or intraoperative cholangiography and ultrasound will reveal in most cases all the secrets of the intraparenchymal anatomy.

References

1. Strasberg SM (1997) Terminology of liver anatomy and liver resections: coming to grips with hepatic Babel. J Am Coll Surg 184:413–433
2. Cantlie J (1897) On a new arrangement of the right and left lobes of the liver. Proc Anat Soc Great Britain Ireland 32:4–9
3. McIndoe AH, Counseler VS (1927) A report on the bilaterality of the liver. Arch Surg 15:589–612
4. Hjortsjö CH (1951) The topography of the intrahepatic duct systems. Acta Anat 1951; 11:599–615
5. Healey JE, Schroy PC (1953) Anatomy of the biliary ducts within the human liver; analysis of the prevailing pattern of branchings and the major variations of the biliary ducts. Arch Surg 66:599–616
6. Couinaud C (1957) Le foie. In: Etudes anatomique et chirurgicales. Paris, Masson
7. Couinaud C (1999) Liver anatomy: portal (and suprahepatic) or biliary segmentation. Dig Surg 16:459–467
8. Henderson JM, Heymsfield SB, Horowitz J, Kutner MH (1981) Measurement of liver and spleen volume by computed tomography. Radiology 141:525–527
9. Kawasaki S, Makuuchi M, Matsunami H et al (1993) Preoperative measurement of segmental liver volume of donors for living-related liver transplantation. Hepatology 18:1115–1120
10. Hiatt JR, Gabbay J, Busuttil RW (1994) Surgical anatomy of the hepatic arteries in 1000 cases. Ann Surg 220:50–52
11. Imamura H, Makuuchi M, Sakamoto Y et al (2000) Anatomical pitfalls in living donor liver transplantation. J Hepatobiliary Pancreat Surg 7:380–394
12. Couinaud C, Houssin D (1991) Controlled partition of the liver for transplantation. Anatomical limitations. Paris
13. Scheuerlein H, Köckerling F (1999) Anatomie der Leber. In: Köckerling F, Waclawiczek HW (eds) Leberchirurgie. Barth, Leipzig
14. Smadja C, Blumgart LH (1994) The biliary tract and the anatomy of biliary exposure. In: Blumgart LH (ed) Surgery of the Liver and Biliary Tract, Vol. I. Churchill Livingstone, Edinburgh
15. Northover JMA, Terblanche J (1979) A new look at the arterial blood supply of the bile duct in man and its surgical implications. Br J Surg 66:379–384
16. Stapleton GN, Hickman R, Terblanche J (1998) Blood supply of the right and left hepatic ducts. Br J Surg 85:202–207
17. Delattre, J-F, Avisse C, Flament J-B (2000) Anatomic basis of hepatic surgery. Surg Clin North Am 80:345–362
18. Broelsch CE, Kremer K, Lüdinghausen M (1993) Leber. In: Chirurgische Operationslehre, Bd. 5. Thieme, Stuttgart
19. Murata S, Itai Y, Asato M, et al. (1995) Effects of temporary occlusion of the hepatic vein on dual blood supply in the liver: evaluation with spiral CT. Radiology 197:351–356
20. Nakamura S, Tsuzuki T (1981) Surgical anatomy of the hepatic veins and the inferior vena cava. Surg Gynecol Obstet 152:43–50

2.2 Consequences of anatomy for the split liver surgeon

D.C. Broering, J. Schulte am Esch, and X. Rogiers

■ Introduction

Splitting the liver into two functional grafts serves to counteract the increasing discrepancy of available liver grafts and patients with terminal liver disease awaiting a life-saving transplantation. During splitting it is very important to keep the quality of the individual graft. Therefore the two grafts derived from one liver need to provide two major features: *appropriate volume* and *appropriate function* relative to the needs of the recipients. This implicates well performed matching of the split graft and recipient. If a left lateral splitting technique is chosen, the left lateral lobe of a adult cadaveric liver is most suitable for children weighing not more than 30 kg.

The extended right split usually provides sufficient volume for large adults up to about 85 kg and can be allocated like a full size liver. Utilizing the full-right full-left splitting technique delivers two medium-sized grafts. The right lobe adequately supports medium adults between 60 to 80 kg of bodyweight, the left small patients with 40 to 60 kg of bodyweight.

In our experience there are five major technical aspects with decreasing impact on adequate function of the split liver graft:

Sufficient venous drainage of *all* segments, grafted
Preservation of bilary vascularization
Appropriate portal perfusion
Physiologic arterial perfusion of *all* segments
Anatomical resection lines during transsection

Some peculiar features of liver anatomy will be addressed that can be crucial for preserving the physiological vascularization and bilary drainage during split liver transplantation.

■ Left lateral splitting for one child and one adult recipient

In general the left liver is more constant regarding anatomical variations compared to the more variant anatomy in the right lobe. Therefore, the more you stay on the left, the fewer anatomical variants that will be seen.

Furthermore, during left lateral splitting, the main vascular hepatic pedicle can stay untouched, and the extended right lobe can be transplanted like a whole organ.

Venous drainage

Anatomical variations of intrahepatic veins are frequently present. These may require individual steps in the splitting procedure in order to assure optimal venous drainage. It is crucial to take any measures to provide optimal venous outflow of all segments to prevent hemorrhagic necrosis. Therefore, all efforts should be made to keep the hepatic veins as much as possible. Prior to the splitting procedure, a careful exploration of the graft is essential to identify variations and to plan the individual steps ahead. The exploration of the venous anatomy can be done during *ex situ* splitting by probing of the veins on the backtable, and during *in situ* splitting with intraoperative ultrasound of the donor liver.

Left hepatic vein

In most of the cases, the left hepatic vein joins the middle hepatic vein extrahepatically, thus forming the common trunk entering the antero-left surface of the inferior vena cava [1] (Fig. 1). But in about 5–10% of livers,

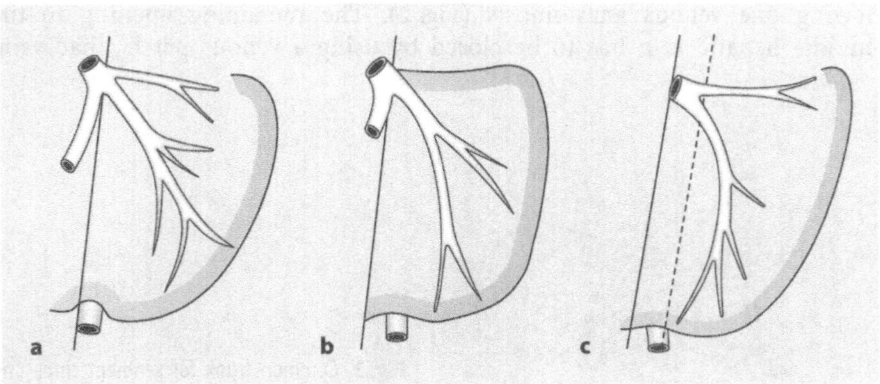

Fig. 1. Frequent variations of the left hepatic veins. The black line illustrates the appropriate line of parenchymal transsection and site of transsection of the left hepatic vein. **a** Common anatomical situation with a short trunk of the left hepatic vein after joining of a small subcapsular segment II vein and the main vein for segments II and III. **b** Long trunk of the left hepatic vein. **c** Large posterior branch of left lateral liver lobe and subcapsular vein joining main left hepatic vein just before entering the common trunk. The broken line is illustration the wrong line of transsection. Moving of the transsection line to the right results in one opening of the left hepatic vein (black line)

they can enter the vena cava separately. In most anatomic situations (>90%) extrahepatic isolation of the left hepatic vein is easily feasible. The diameter of the extrahepatic portion of the left hepatic vein is around 10 mm [2]. A smaller diameter of the left hepatic vein (<7 mm) is sufficient reason to suspict separate drainage of the segment III vein into the middle hepatic vein.

Variations of the segment II and III veins within the left lateral lobe are usually of less surgical consequence for left lateral splitting. A significant posterior subcapsular segment II vein draining separately into the common trunk or inferior vena cava is of surgical consequence (Fig. 1 c). In this situation the transsection line of the left hepatic vein should move as much as possible to the right without narrowing the middle hepatic vein to achieve one opening for anastomosis. If two separated venous stumps can be seen on the resection plane after dividing of the left hepatic vein(s), these veins should be anastomosed on the backtable to recreate one venous opening, thus, allowing only one venous anastomosis during implantation.

A second important anatomical variation is the drainage of the segment III vein into the middle hepatic vein (Fig. 2). Early detection of this variation is especially important during *in situ* splitting, since opening of this vein during parenchymal division results in severe bleeding. Therefore it is important to perform a meticulous parenchymal division technique, thus, allowing identification of this anatomic variation intraoperatively. After appropriate identification of this variation during *in situ* splitting, it is useful to continue the parenchymal division on the backtable after harvesting of the whole liver and perfusion in the regular manner. The division of the common trunk should end up with a nice patch on the left side, thus, allowing one venous anastomosis (Fig. 2). The remaining opening in the middle hepatic vein has to be closed by using a venous patch (iliac vein,

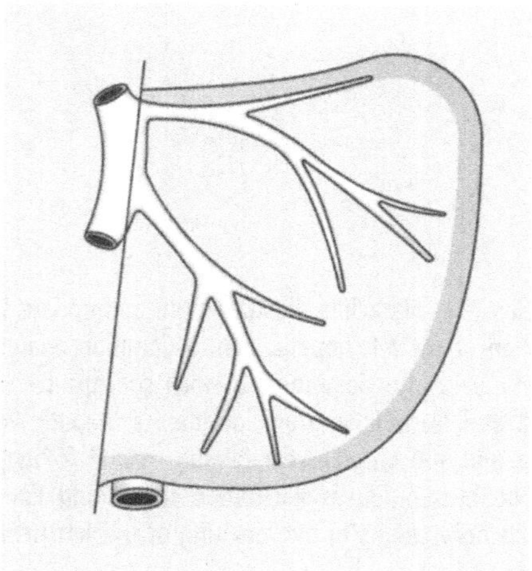

Fig. 2. Common trunk for segment three and middle hepatic vein. The black line indicates the appropriate site of transsection of the parenchyma and the middle hepatic vein, thus providing patches on both grafts for anastomosis with the recipient cava. The remaining defect of the middle hepatic vein can be easily closed with a patch from the donor caval vein to avoid any narrowing of the outflow of middle hepatic vein

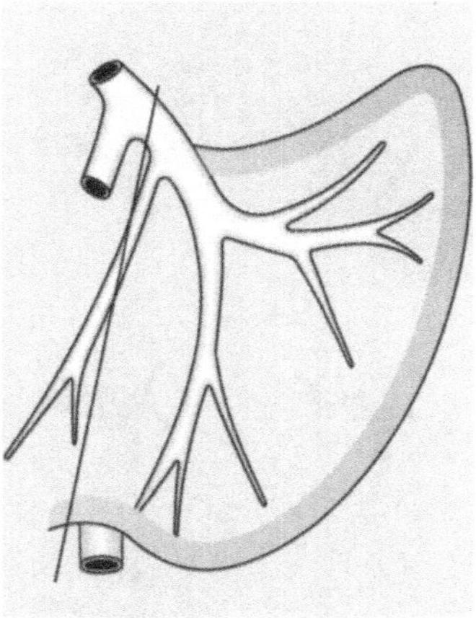

Fig. 3. Fissural vein: partial drainage of a segment IV vein into the left hepatic vein. This vein can usually be divided during parenchymal transsection, because venous collateralization within segment IV and drainage via the middle hepatic vein is always present

caval vein) to avoid outflow obstruction of segment IV and the right medial segments (V, VIII).

In some patients along the umbilical fissure, a small hepatic vein, draining parts of segment IV (Fig. 3) may be found. This fissural vein crosses the umbilical fissure, thus, draining via the segment III vein and left hepatic vein into the common trunk. This vein is of no surgical consequence for left lateral splitting and can be discarded during parenchymal division. The real challenge is to distinguish during parenchymal transsection between a segment III vein, which should be preserved, and a fissural vein. Fissural veins cross the umbilical fissure from right inferior to left superior, compared to segment III veins draining into the middle hepatic vein which cross from left inferior to right superior.

Biliary tract

During initial period of left lateral split liver transplantation many groups performed isolation of the main left hepatic duct next to the main bile duct bifurcation for harvesting of the left lateral lobe to create a nice bile duct stump at the left lateral lob for anastomosis in the recipient. This technique was associated with a high rate of biliary complications on both grafts due to the following reasons [3]. First, leaving a long stump of the left bile duct with the left lateral graft results in a high risk of ischemic necrosis of the bile duct due to damaging of the parabiliary vascular plexus during isolation of the left bile duct [4]. Second, the high incidence of biliary complications was due to the high prevalence of damaging the segment I and IV bile duct(s) of the right extended lobe. After moving the transsection line to the left at the umbilical fissure behind the umbilical portion of

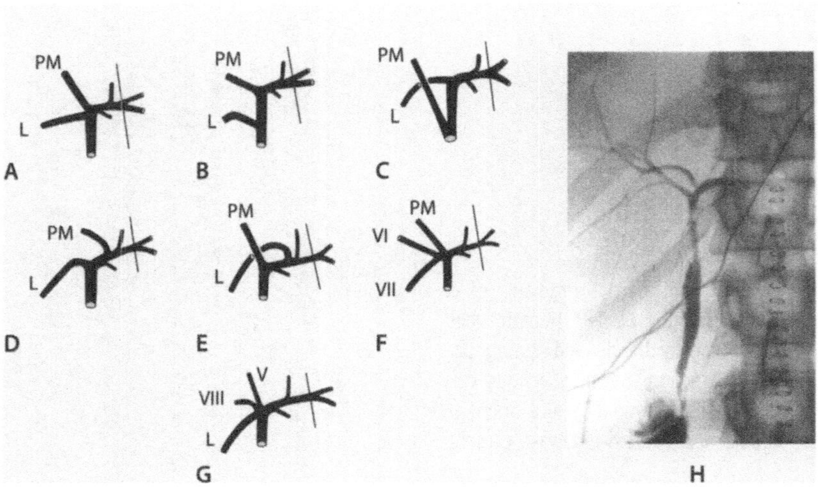

Fig. 4. Variations of biliary anatomy within the right liver lobe [2]. If the cutting line of the umbilical plate stays behind the umbilical portion of the left portal vein at the umbilical fissure (dotted line), the biliary system of the right extended graft will not be compromised (**A–G**). The dotted line indicates the umbilical fissure, the line of transsection of the umbilical plate. *PM* paramedian segments of the right lobe (segments V and VIII); *L* Lateral segments of the right lobe (segments VI and VII). **H** Postoperative t-tube cholangiography 7 days after implantation of a right extended graft (segments I, IV to VIII) with end-to-end anastomosis of the common bile ducts. The right lateral bile duct arises from the left main bile duct (see also Fig. 4D) and has not been affected by the left lateral split technique

the left portal vein and avoiding any dissection at the umbilical plate, the incidence of biliary complications dropped [5, 6].

Variations of the bile ducts are more frequent in the right lobe compared with the left lobe. Therefore moving of the transsection plane to the left behind the left main portal vein reduces the risk of damaging important bile ducts of the right extended graft. In regular anatomy, the risk of narrowing of segment I and segment IV bile ducts is significantly lower if the plane of division of the umbilical plate is at the umbilical fissure, without compromising safety of reconstruction of biliary drainage of the graft after implantation. Intraoperative cholangiography is usually not necessary during left lateral liver splitting. If anatomical variations of the biliary system are present at the hilum or within the right lobe, these atypical bile ducts are also not interfered with using this technique of bile duct transsection (Fig. 4). Figure 4 H illustrates a postoperative cholangiography 7 days after implantation of a right extended graft (segment I, IV to VIII) derived from left lateral *in situ* splitting. The right lateral bile duct drains into the left main bile duct, but is not narrowed by the splitting procedure.

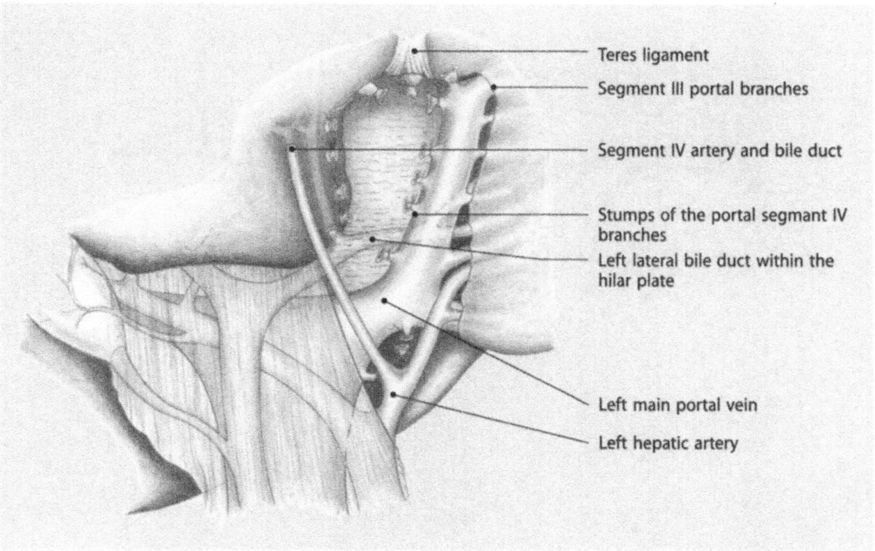

Fig. 5. Anatomic situation after dissection of the portal branches to segment IV. The left hilar plate behind the left portal vein is exposed. In most cases the bile duct(s) within the hilar plate can be seen

There are only very rare anatomical variations of the bile ducts in which a left lateral splitting is not possible, e.g., the main bile duct bifurcation is located behind the left portal vein.

In most instances (55%) the union of segment II and III ducts to form the left lateral bile duct is located at the umbilical fissure within the umbilical plate [7] (Fig. 5). Therefore, one goal during transsection of the umbilical plate is to achieve one opening for biliary anastomosis, thus, minimizing the risk of biliary complications in the recipient of the left lateral graft. In 30% of the donor livers the union of segment II and III is located left to the umbilical fissure [7]. Considering this anatomical data, two bile ducts on the left lateral graft should results in only 15% of the cases. Figure 6 illustrates different types of biliary anatomy at the umbilical fissure and the consequences for the split liver surgeon.

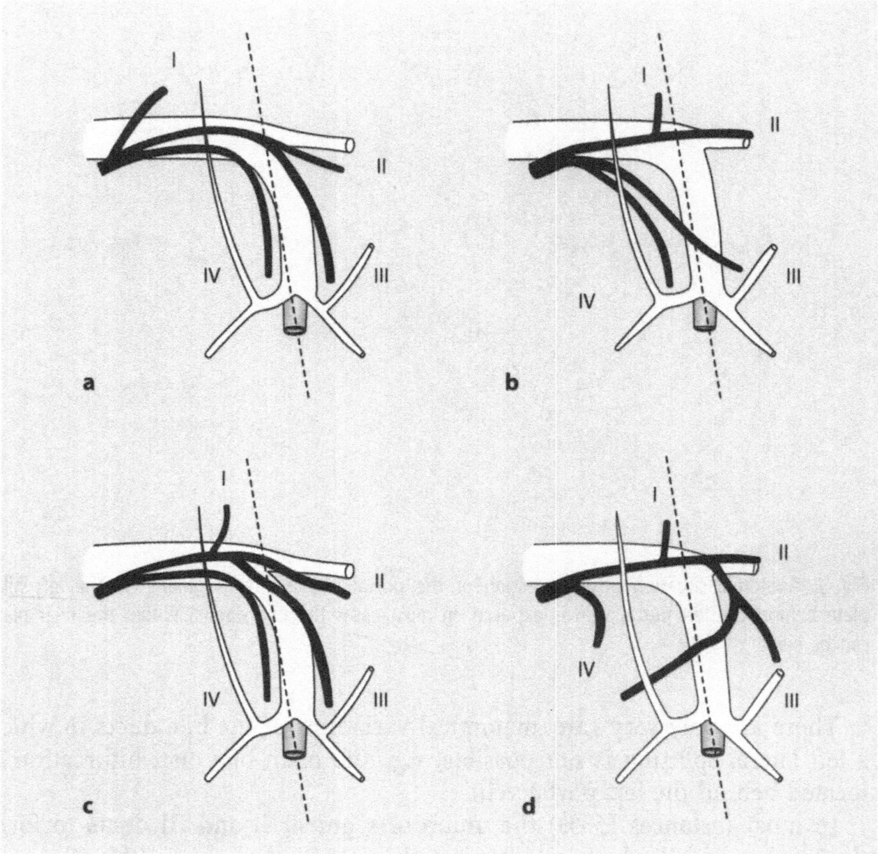

Fig. 6. Variations of the course of the left bile ducts within the umbilical plate in relation to the umbilical portion of the left portal vein and the umbilical fissure (dotted line) [2]. **a** Union of segment II and III bile duct at the umbilical fissure resulting in one opening for anastomosis at the stump of the hilar plate. **b** Late (central or right) union of segment II and III bile duct. In addition confluence of segment IV and III bile duct before conjunction with segment II bile duct. **c** Union of the segment II and three bile duct medial to the umbilical fissure resulting in two separate openings for segment II and III bile ducts. Moving to the right with the transsection line of the umbilical plate would result in damaging segment I and (or) segment IV bile duct. **d** Segment IV bile duct crosses the umbilical fissure, thus, draining into segment III bile duct. This rare variation is no contraindication for left lateral splitting, since in our experience additional segment IV bile ducts can be found

Portal vein

Embryology of the portal vein is first established; then, arteries and biliary ducts invade the liver following approximately the portal branches. Thus, intrahepatic portal venous variations can be seen in approximately 20% of the population [8, 9]. In the vast majority of cases they consist, in decreas-

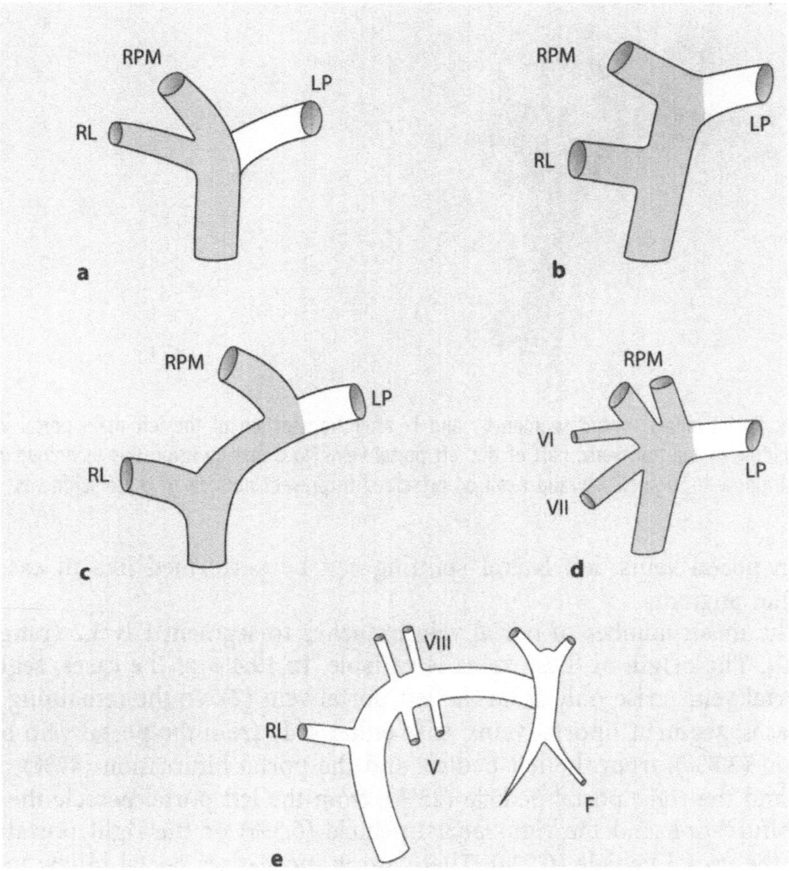

Fig. 7. Variations of the right portal veins if the right portal vein is missing (*Modified from C. Couinaud, Surgery of the Liver Revisited (1989) [2]).* Shaded area: portal system, which stays with the right lobe. White: portal system, which stays with the left lateral lobe. **a** Portal trifurcation (8%), **b** Caudal origin of the right lateral vein (RL) (10%), **c** Right paramedian portal vein (RPM) from left main portal vein (2.7%), **d** Duplication of the RPM and RL (0.9%), **e** Contraindication for split liver transplantation in a case of a missing main portal vein bifurcation (0.9%)

ing order of frequency, of a trifurcation of the main portal vein (Fig. 7 a), a posterior segmental branch arising from the main portal vein (Fig. 7 b), and a right anterior segmental branch arising from the left portal vein (Fig. 7 c).

The rare absence of a portal vein bifurcation (absence of left portal vein, Fig. 7 e) is a contraindication for left lateral splitting. In the case of a right paramedian portal vein coming from the left vein (Fig. 7 c), transsection of the left portal vein has to move to the left to avoid narrowing of the portal vein supplying segments V and VIII. In the remaining variations of the

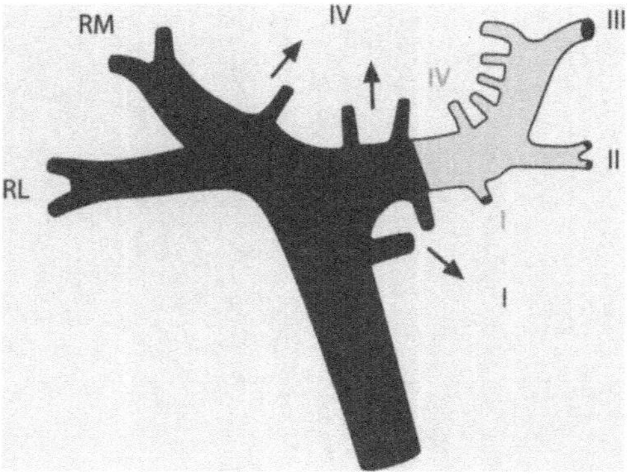

Fig. 8. Portal inflow toward segments I and IV after transsection of the left main portal vein in the middle of the transverse part of the left portal vein. Note that by using this technique, partial portal inflow to segments IV and I can be preserved to prevent necrosis of these segments

main portal veins, left lateral splitting can be performed like in cases of regular anatomy.

The mean number of portal vein branches to segment I is 3.2 (range 1–6) [2]. The origin of these veins is variable. In 19.4% of the cases, segment I portal veins arise only from the left portal vein (2). In the remaining 80% of cases, segment I portal veins arise either only from the portal vein bifurcation (2.8%), from the left pedicle and the portal bifurcation (47%), from left and the right portal pedicle (23%), from the left portal pedicle the portal bifurcation and the right portal pedicle (6.5%) or the right portal vein and the portal pedicle (0.9%). Therefore in most cases portal inflow to segment I can be preserved despite harvesting of the left main portal vein with the left lateral graft. In the case of portal segment I branches arising only from the left portal vein, the line of transsection of the left portal vein can be moved to the left to preserve the first one or two portal segment I veins (Fig. 8).

The portal vein inflow to segment IV varies greatly. The majority of the portal inflow to segment IV is accomplished from left umbilical portion of the left portal vein. Since this vein stays with the left lateral graft, all segment IV veins arising from umbilical portion of the left portal vein have to be transsected. But in most cases there are additional portal vein branches to segment IV from the portal vein bifurcation and the right portal vein. By preserving these veins and moving the transsection line to the left, thus, with the additional preservation of segment IV portal veins (Fig. 8), partial portal inflow to segment IV can be preserved.

Hepatic artery

The main goal during dissection of the hepatic artery is to explore the individual arterial anatomy of the donor and to find the correct position for separation of the arterial supply of both grafts. The arterial blood supply of every segment of the two grafts should be maintained to avoid diminished function or segmental necrosis of the grafts.

Variations of the hepatic artery are frequent. Only 50–70% of livers present with "normal" anatomy [10, 11]. A replaced artery can be found in 30%. The left artery is featured with more complex variations if contrasted with the right hepatic artery.

Variations of the hepatic artery are not considered contraindications for splitting, but they do determine the site of transsection of the artery and the number of anastomosis, which have to be performed for complete arterial reperfusion of both grafts. In contrast, malformations of the hepatic artery (aneurysma, etc.) have to be considered as contraindications for splitting.

If the left main hepatic artery comes from the left gastric artery (10 to 15%), this artery is usually very long and has a nice diameter for anastomosis in the recipient. This artery can be dissected down to the celiac trunk including the left gastric artery. In this situation, the celiac trunk itself usually stays with the right graft. In most instances the very small regular left hepatic artery (<2 mm) coming from the proper hepatic artery can be discarded. But if the diameter of this artery reaches 2 mm and arterial backflow after implantation is not convincing, this artery should also be anastomosed in the recipient.

A replaced right hepatic artery (15%), coming from the superior mesenteric artery, is of less consequence for left lateral splitting. Dissection and transsection of the left hepatic artery has to be performed like in cases of regular anatomy. In this situation, the segment IV artery arises mostly from the proper hepatic artery and can stay in continuity with the celiac trunk.

The rare arterial variation of a completely displaced hepatic artery arising from the superior mesenteric artery (2%) also has no consequences for left lateral splitting.

Since the majority of the portal blood supply toward segment IV has to be sacrificed, arterial supply of segment IV determines survival of this segment. Therefore, every effort should be given to preserve the segment IV artery during dissection of the left portal vein without compromising the arterial inflow toward the left lateral liver lobe.

In most of the cases, the median hepatic artery (segment IV) arises from the left hepatic artery (Fig. 9 a). In this situation the left hepatic artery can be transsected distally to the origin of the segment IV artery, if the diameter of the left hepatic artery is still more than 2 mm.

If there is a trifurcation of the right, middle and left hepatic artery the left artery should be transsected without compromising the inflow toward segment IV.

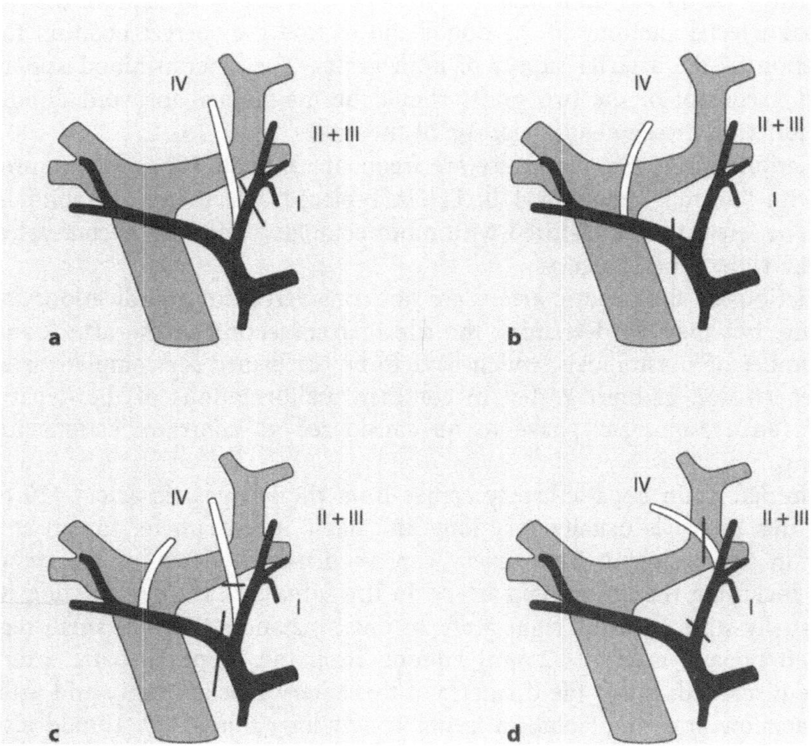

Fig. 9. Different variations of arterial blood supply toward segment IV. Black lines illustrate the site of transsection of the arteries to achieve appropriate inflow toward both grafts

If the segment IV artery arises very distally from the left hepatic artery (Fig. 9d), the segment IV artery has to be cut down and can be anastomosed on the backtable to the stump of the left hepatic artery with 8/0 PDS in an end-to-end fashion using magnifying loops, if the celiac trunk stays in continuity with the right graft.

In some patients the segment IV artery arises only from the right hepatic artery (Fig. 9b); thus, the celiac trunk should stay with the left graft, because the diameter of the right hepatic artery is larger than that of the left hepatic artery, making anastomosis of the left graft safer.

If arterial blood supply of segment IV is realized via the left and right hepatic artery (Fig. 9c), the cutting points can be chosen as in exclusively right supplied livers (Fig. 9b).

■ Full right – full left splitting

Full right – full left splitting means splitting of the liver along the line of Cantilie resulting in one full right lobe (segment V to VIII) and one full left lobe (segment I to IV). With this technique, the splitting surgeon can usually create two medium-sized grafts for implantation. Due to the large resection plane in the middle of the liver, the splitting surgeon is faced with special anatomical problems.

Hepatic veins

If the middle hepatic vein stays with the full left graft, venous drainage of segment II to IV is achieved via the middle and left hepatic veins joining as a common trunk to drain into the caval vein. Since segment I drains directly into the caval vein, this segment loses venous outflow if the caval vein stays with the right graft. First attempts of transplantation of left grafts (segment II to IV) without the caval vein showed a high percentage of venous outflow problems due to kinking at the anastomosis between the recipients caval vein and the common trunk of the graft. Therefore, groups have started to leave the caval vein with the left graft to avoid the kinking

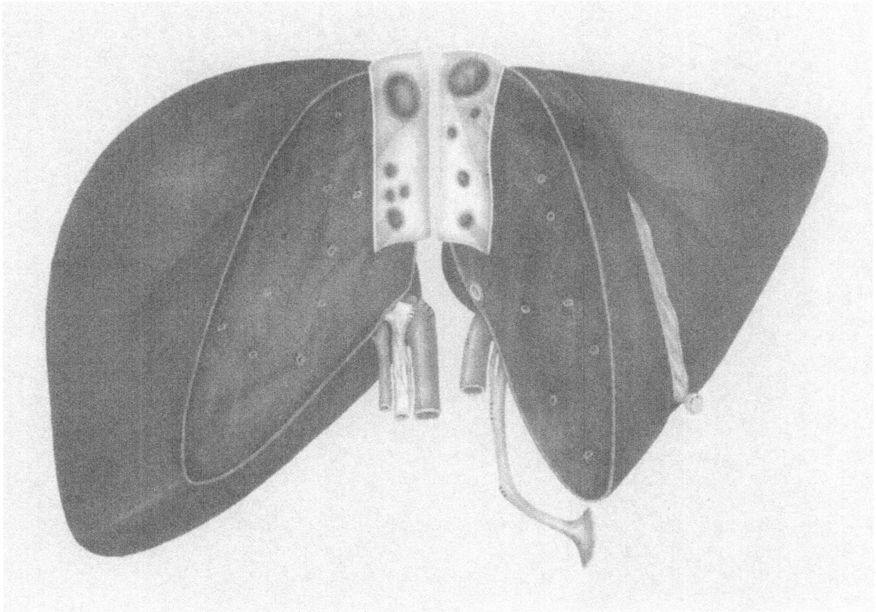

Fig. 10. Split cava technique: splitting the vena cava results in two large patches on both grafts. The right patch at the right graft (segments V to VIII) includes the right hepatic vein and retrohepatic veins draining dorsal parts of the right liver. The patch on the left graft (segments I to IV) includes the common trunk and the veins of segment I, draining directly into the caval vein

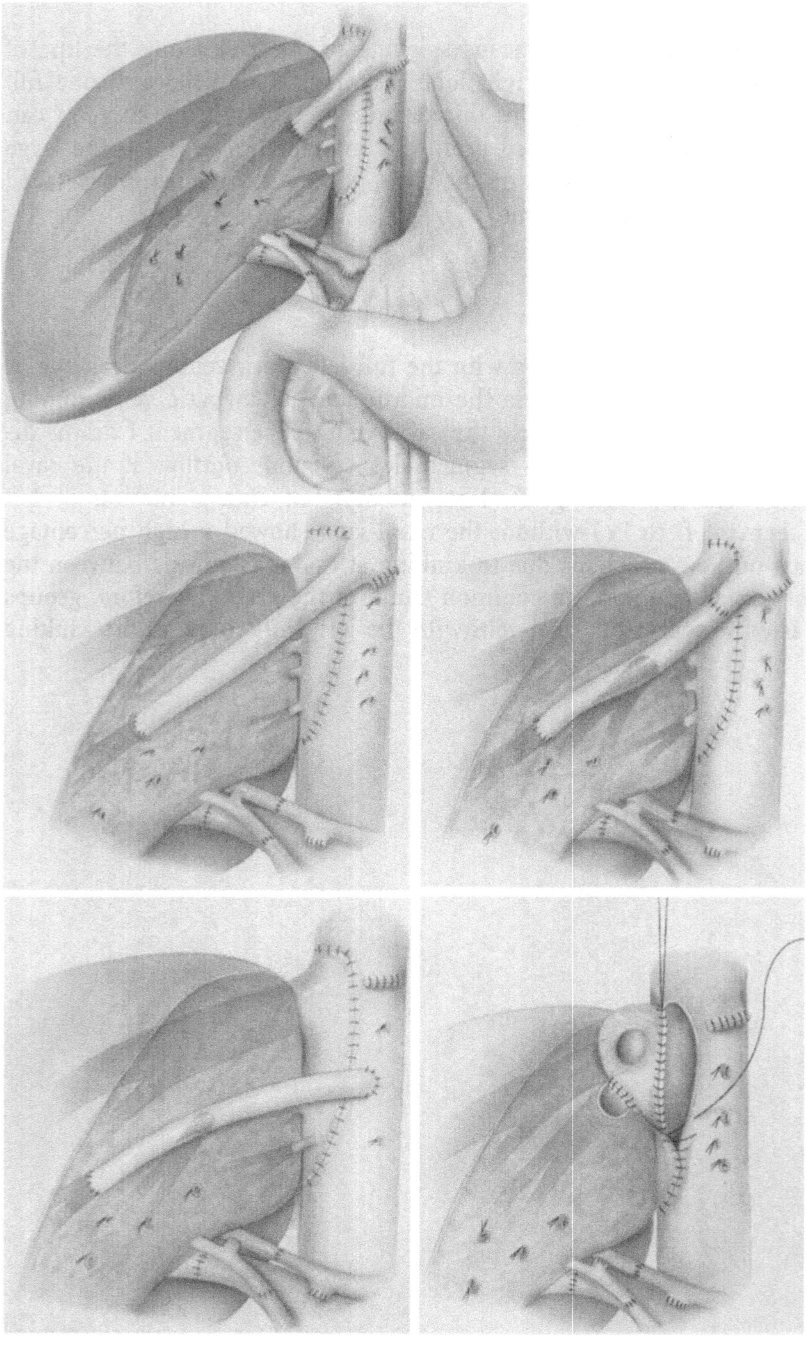

Fig. 11. Different types of reconstruction of venous outflow of segments V and VIII

of the venouse anastomosis and to also allow easy transplantation of segment I. By leaving the caval vein with left graft, the right graft loses the venous outflow via the short retrohepatic veins draining directly into the caval vein. In addition, the anastomosis of the right hepatic vein carries the risk of kinking or narrowing at the anastomosis. To overcome these problems on both grafts, we developed the split cava technique to share the caval vein between both grafts [12] (Fig. 10).

With this technique, the venous outflow of segment I stays in continuity with the left half of the caval vein and the conjunction of the common trunk with the caval vein can be preserved, thus allowing a large side-to-side anastomosis between the recipient's caval vein and the caval patch on the left graft, which reduces the risk of kinking of the venous anastomosis. The retrohepatic short veins remains with the right half of the caval vein, thus making anastomosis of larger retrohepatic vein unnecessary. The second advantage for the right graft is that anastomosis of the right caval patch, compared to the end-to-side anastomosis of the right hepatic vein and the vena cava is much easier and saver. The only problem, which stays unsolved with the split cava technique, is the possible congestion of segments V and VIII, if these segments are mainly drained via the middle hepatic vein.

To overcome this problem, we perform anastomosis of the stumps of segment V and VIII veins (more than 5 mm in diameter) at the resection plane on the backtable in an end-to-side fashion with a iliac vein of the donor, which itself has to be anastomosed in the recipient either directly with the recipients caval vein or the stump of the recipients middle hepatic vein. Fig. 11 illustrates various techniques of reconstruction of segment V and VIII veins during full right – full left splitting.

With these two techniques (split cava technique and reconstruction of segment V and VIII veins), the problem of anatomical variations and venous outflow can be considered resolved.

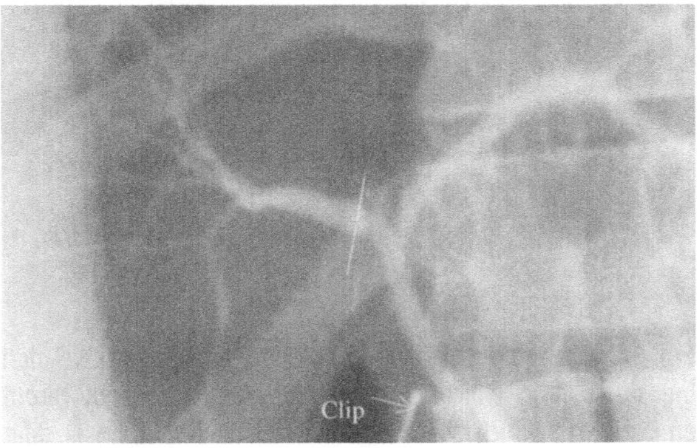

Fig. 12. Intraoperative cholangiography of the donor liver during *in situ* full right – full left splitting. Segment I bile duct arise from the right main bile duct; therefore, the common bile duct stays with the left graft. Black line: Recommended site of transsection of the right bile duct. The clip marks the beginning of the main right bile duct

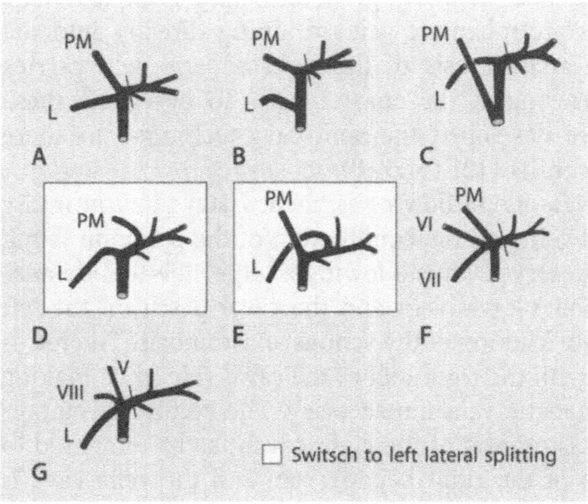

Fig. 13. Managing of variations of right biliary anatomy during full right – full left splitting. Black lines are illustrating site of transsection of the bile duct

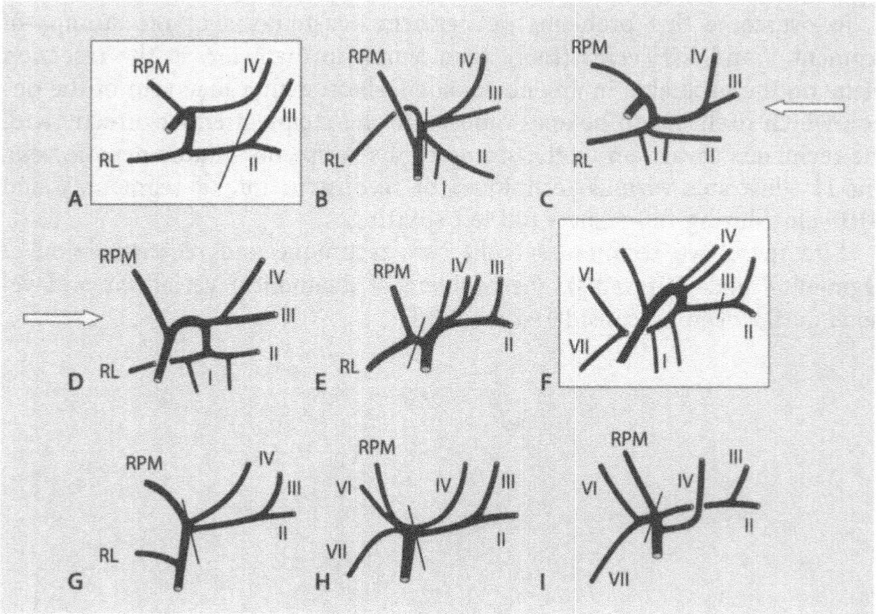

Fig. 14. Managing of left-sided bile duct variations in full right – full left splitting. Arrows indicating situation in which a splitting of the liver is not recommended. Rectangles indicate biliary anomalies in which switching to left lateral splitting is safer. Black lines: site of transsection of the bile duct

Bile ducts

Anatomic variability of bile ducts, especially within the right lobe and at the hilum, is the most demanding problem in full right - full left splitting. The main advantage over living-donor liver transplantation using either the full right or full left lobe, is that the splitting surgeon can decide upon individual anatomy at which graft the common bile duct should remain. Therefore the splitting surgeon has to examine the bile duct anatomy clinically and with intraoperative cholangiography prior to deciding whether a full right - full left split is meaningful and at which graft the common bile duct should stay.

If intraoperative cholangiography reveals regular anatomy with a long main right bile duct, the common bile duct should remain with the left graft. To find the right point of division of the right main bile duct, a metallic clip is placed during intraoperative cholangiography (Fig. 12).

In cases of complex biliary variations at the right biliary tree, the common bile duct should stay either with the right graft (Fig. 13 a–c, f, g) or the splitting surgeon should switch to a left lateral splitting technique (Fig. 13 d, e) to minimize the risk of postoperative biliary complications.

If during intraoperative cholangiography complex variations within both livers are observed, splitting has to cease in selected cases (Fig. 14 c and d). In some situations switching to a left lateral splitting technique is recommended (Fig. 14 a and f).

Portal vein

Sharing of the portal vein between the two grafts during full right - full left splitting is usually easily feasible. In regular anatomy, the question were the main portal vein should stay, depends on the individual recipient's conditions. If significant portal segment IV branches arise from the right main portal vein, the transsection line of the right portal vein has move to the right as described for living-donor right lobe grafting [13]. Variations of the right portal venous system usually lead to leaving the main portal vein with the right graft (Fig. 7). The absence of the left portal vein is also a contraindication for full right - full left splitting.

Hepatic artery

Sharing of the hepatic artery is normally also easily feasible in full right - full left splitting. The segment IV artery, which is very important for the left graft, has to remain with the left hepatic artery and in most instances with the celiac trunk. If the segment IV artery arises from the right hepatic artery, the side of transsection of the right hepatic artery has to move to the right, as described for portal vein transsection.

■ Conclusions

Choosing anatomical resection lines yield in both fewer biliary complications and lower blood loss during parenchymal dissection. Respecting and preserving the venous outflow is vital. Careful handling of the parabiliary vascular plexus is crucial in order to prevent bile duct necrosis. Portal and arterial reconstruction is almost always possible (magnifying glasses) and should be performed. The less invasive split line is the left lateral. Unfortunately, not every liver is splitable. Be aware of main anatomic variants.

■ References

1. Sharma D, Deshmukh A, Raina VK (2001) Surgical anatomy of retrohepatic inferior vena cava and hepatic veins: a quantitative assessment. Indian J Gastroenterol 20(4):136–139
2. Couinaud C (1989) Surgical Anatomy of the Liver Revisited, Paris
3. Broelsch CE, Emond JC, Whitington PF, Thistlethwaite JR, Baker AL, Lichtor JL (1990) Application of reduced-size liver transplants as split grafts, auxiliary orthotopic grafts, and living related segmental transplants. Ann Surg 212(3): 368–3675; discussion 375–377
4. Stapleton GN, Hickman R, Terblanche J (1998) Blood supply of the right and left hepatic ducts. Br J Surg 85(2):202–207
5. Rogiers X, Malago M, Gawad K, Jauch KW, Olausson M, Knoefel WT, Gundlach M, Bassas A, Fischer L, Sterneck M, Burdelski M, Broelsch CE (1996) In situ splitting of cadaveric livers. The ultimate expansion of a limited donor pool. Ann Surg 224(3):331–339; discussion 339–341
6. Broering DC, Mueller L, Ganschow R, Kim JS, Achilles EG, Schafer H, Gundlach M, Fischer L, Sterneck M, Hillert C, Helmke K, Izbicki JR, Burdelski M, Rogiers X (2001). Is there still a need for living-related liver transplantation in children? Ann Surg 234(6):713–721; discussion 721–722
7. Reichert PR, Renz JF, D'Albuquerque LA, Rosenthal P, Lim RC, Roberts JP, Ascher NL, Emond JC (2000). Surgical anatomy of the left lateral segment as applied to living-donor and split-liver transplantation: a clinicopathologic study. Ann Surg 232(5):658–664
8. Atri M, Bret PM, Fraser-Hill MA (1992) Intrahepatic portal venous variations: prevalence with US. Radiology 184:157–158
9. Couinaud C (ed) The Liver: Anatomic and Surgical Studies. Masson, Paris, pp 71–118
10. Michels NA (1966) Newer anatomy of the liver and its variation in blood supply and collateral circulation. Am J Surg 112:337–346
11. Y. Kawarada B, Das C, Taoka H (2000) Anatomy of the hepatic hilar area: the plate system. J Hepatobiliary Pancreat Surg 7:580–586
12. Gundlach M, Broering D, Topp S, Sterneck M, Rogiers X (2000) Split-cava technique: liver splitting for two adult recipients. Liver Transpl 6(6):703–706
13. Marcos A (2000) Right lobe living donor liver transplantation: a review. Liver Transpl 6(1):3–20

2.3 H.J. Schlitt

Which liver is splitable?

Liver splitting for transplantation purposes is based on four major premises:

- the lobular anatomic structure of the liver that allows for separation of functionally independent subunits;
- the high functional reserve of a healthy liver that makes 30–40% of the standard organ mass sufficient for life support;
- the strong regenerative capacity which generally enables growth of the transplanted organ part to reach a normal liver mass within a few weeks; and
- the increasing knowledge and skill of liver transplant surgeons. Considering these facts in light of the limited number of donor organs available, liver splitting should be performed whenever possible in order to increase the number of transplantable organ parts.

Successful liver splitting and subsequent split liver transplantation, however, requires thorough consideration and evaluation whenever an organ donor is available. The decision about whether or not to split a given donor liver – and if yes whether to do it *in situ* or *ex situ* – depends on a number of variables which have different degrees of impact on the decision making. These variables include formal donor-related data, the given anatomic situation, the macroscopic appearance of the liver, the size and clinical state of the potential recipients, the availability of an experienced surgeon, and a number of other logistic aspects (Table 1).

Table 1. Factors influencing the decision about splitting

Donor parameters: age, time on ICU, Na^+, ASAT, γGT, cause of death, hemodynamic stability
Intraoperative parameters: macroscopic appearance, anatomic variants
Logistic parameters: *in situ/ex situ* splitting, donor hospital, availability of experienced surgeon
Recipient parameters: HU situation/critical recipient, recipient size/weight

Table 2. Optimal donor parameters for liver splitting

■ Young, healthy donor (< 40(–50) years of age)
■ No history of liver disease/damage
■ Normal liver enzymes (ASAT, ALAT, γGT)
■ Short ICU time (≤2 days)
■ Hemodynamic stability
■ Macroscopically normal liver

Clearly, the ideal liver for splitting (Table 2) would be from a young donor with no history of liver disease or damage, with normal liver enzymes (particularly the γ-glutamyl-transpeptidase (γGT)), and short intensive care (ICU) time who is hemodynamically stable before and during the donor operation. Macroscopically, the liver should have a soft consistency, be sharp-edged, and preferably have a large left-lateral lobe (unless the recipient of this part is a very small child); a separate left hepatic artery would be welcome. For optimal logistics, this donor should be available in the transplant center itself to have optimal conditions for *in situ* splitting. Unfortunately, these criteria are fulfilled only by a small minority of the currently available organ donors so that in clinical practice compromises are frquently necessary.

In our center the recent series of liver splitting from 1996 to 1999 consists of 66 transplants. This includes transplantation of 31 right and 35 left liver parts into 34 adult and 32 pediatric patients. Nine of the split procedures were performed *in situ*; 24 were performed *ex situ*. Retransplantation was required in 10 of the 66 patients (15.2%), mainly for initial non-function of the graft. Eleven of the 66 patients (16.7%) died, and in 3 of these cases initial non-function of the graft was the major cause of death (including one with graft failure after auxiliary transplantation). The donors of livers that had been accepted for splitting had a median age of 27 years, but 10 of them were older than 40, and 3 older than 50 years. About half of the donors were trauma victims while the others had died from spontaneous intracranial hemorrhage. Median time of intensive care treatment was 2 days, but 4 donors had been in the ICU for more than 3 days and one even for 9 days. The majority of donors had normal ASAT levels (< 20 U/l); in 9 donors it was > 30 U/l with a maximum of 175 U/l. The median γGT was 7.5 U/l; only one donor had a γGT above 30 U/l. In 3 donors serum sodium concentration was >160 mmol/l with a maximum of 166; the median sodium level was 149 mmol/l. Positive inotropic support, either high or low dose, was required in almost all organ donors. There was no obvious correlation between donor parameters and the development of initial non-function. The pediatric recipient of a left lateral lobe obtained from our oldest donor (54 years) had prolonged jaundice but over time liver function normalized completely.

Although donor parameters are critical for selecting livers for a splitting procedure, definition of absolute contraindications is difficult. There are, however, several parameters that argue stronlgy against splitting even prior to seeing the liver in the donor. These parameters are high age (>60 years), high serum sodium level (>170 mmol/l), and high γGT (>100 U/l). Moreover, a long ICU treatment of the donor (>5 days) makes the availability of a splitable organ very unlikely. Nevertheless, splitting of livers from such donors may be considered in individual cases after *in situ* evaluation of the organ, but mostly these parameters will be associated with suboptimal organ quality. Particularly if a donor fulfills several of these parameters at the same time, an organ quality suitable for splitting is highly unlikely – although this suboptimal or borderline organ may still be transplantable as a whole.

The most reliable basis for the decision about whether to split or not to split a given donor liver is the intraoperative judgment by the harvesting surgeon. Since splitting requires additional manipulation of the liver – either during harvesting *in situ* or after harvesting *ex situ* – the quality requirements are markedly higher than for whole liver transplantation in order to avoid a high risk of initial graft dysfunction. Therefore, only excellent or very good livers should generally be used for splitting. Intraoperative evaluation of the donor organ is of particular importance not only for evaluation of organ quality but also for assessing the size of the organ and its lobes. If a liver is principally splitable but its anatomy is inadequate for a chosen recipient, selection of an alternative recipient either in the same or in another center should be considered. Anatomic variants of the blood vessels are usually no contraindication for splitting; an aberrant left hepatic artery from the left gastric artery or a separate right hepatic artery from the superior mesenteric artery may even be preferable for the splitting procedure.

Considering the technical and logistical differences of *ex situ* vs. *in situ* splitting, the method used may also have an influence on the decision of whether or not to split a given organ. Since *in situ* splitting is mostly associated with shorter ischemic time and no additional damage due to suboptimal cooling and manipulation during *ex situ* preparation, organs that are not considered adequate for *ex situ* splitting may be successfully splitted with the *in situ* technique. Thus, *in situ* splitting may allow a broader use of donor organs for splitting purposes.

The prospective recipients are also of relevance for the decision about whether or not to split. In an adult high urgency transplant situation, splitting may be contraindicated even if an excellent donor organ is available – in order to provide the critically ill patient with an optimal donor organ and a maximum liver mass. In contrast, in case of high urgency in a pediatric recipient, size reduction of an adult donor organ would be required anyway so that splitting should be performed in most of these cases. In an elective situation, selection of the most suitable recipients should best be done after intraoperative assessment of the donor organ and the absolute size of the respective lobes to be generated by the splitting procedure. If no recipients with an adequate weight are available in a single center then sharing of the liver with another center should be considered.

In clinical practice the decision about whether or not to split a given donor liver is a multistep procedure. The primary selection will be made based on the available data of the donor and may lead to exclusion if one or several of the above mentioned negative predictive criteria are met. With the increasing number of older and non-trauma donors, the relative proportion of "excellent" donors has markedly decreased over the last decade so that currently less than 20% of all donors available in the Eurotransplant area may be suitable for splitting. If all parameters suggest a very good or excellent organ, then the final decision will be based on the intraoperative assessment during the harvesting procedure – with consideration of the potential recipients. In the case that another team performs the harvesting with the intent to do *ex situ* splitting in the transplant center, the decision about the splitting may even be delayed until the liver has been seen and reevaluated at the transplanting center.

Lastly, the decision about whether or not to split a given donor liver depends on logistical issues, e.g., whether the donor center has a surgeon available who is able and willing to do the splitting procedure. Training of transplant surgeons in these techniques is, therefore, an important goal. Alternatively, surgeons from larger centers might be available for performing splitting procedures together with the collegues from the actual donor center. The major problem in this regard, however, is that centers who do not practice pediatric liver transplantation have a no real incentive to support the splitting because it leaves them with a reduced size organ graft for their adult patient that may carry a slightly increased technical risk at transplantation while they have no obvious benefits from sharing part of the liver.

Because of these organizational problems, a large number of potentially splitable donor livers are being lost for this use. Improvement of the current situation, therefore, requires three steps:

- a priori identification of potentially splitable donor livers, i.e., preselection of "very good" donors (e.g., see Table 1);
- creating incentives for smaller centers to cooperate in the splitting activities; and
- development of organizational structures that make liver splitting possible in all locations and at all times.

3 Techniques for splitting the liver

3.1 D. Azoulay and D. Castaing

The Paris technique

Liver transplantation has become the best treatment available today for end-stage liver disease. Since the first successful human orthotopic liver transplant by Thomas Starzl in 1963 [1], many advances in immunosuppression, perioperative care and graft preservation have been necessary to obtain reliable results. Currently the main concern in liver transplantation is organ shortage. To overcome this restraint, liver surgeons have explored several possibilities [2]. Thus, through an extensive knowledge of the liver anatomy, the use of one graft for two recipients (the so-called split technique) has become a major breakthrough. Splitting the liver is now routinely performed either *in situ* or once explanted, with results comparable to those using a whole liver. The following description is the technique of *ex situ* split liver transplantation we have developed at the Paul Brousse Hospital in Paris.

■ Graft evaluation and preparation

Hepatectomy in the donor is performed using the *en bloc* rapid technique of Starzl [3]. To avoid warm ischemia, the liver is cooled by infusion of University of Wisconsin unpreservation solution. Assessment of the quality of the graft is as important as the selection of the recipients for the two grafts. The selection of the recipient of the left graft is especially important.

The liver is prepared on the "back table". An ice bath of UW solution maintains the liver temperature at less than 4 °C in the meantime, while the operating room temperature is maintained at 10 °C. The procedure is carried out as for a whole graft [3]. The cystic duct is ligated after the cholecystectomy, to insure that there is no leak during the cholangiography that we perform systematically. At this stage, absence of portal bifurcation, the only absolute contraindication to splitting the liver [4], is checked using a metal cannula to probe the portal trunk.

We consider predissection cholangiography and arteriography indispensable for precise delineation of the intra-hepatic distribution of the glissonian pedicles since unrecocognized distorted anatomy may result in disastrous consequences [5]. This does not increase morbidity, nor lengthen the operating time.

A radiograph is done after the injection of pure contrast media (Radioselectan® 76%, Schering SA, Lys-les-lannoy, France) into the distal bile duct, through a 8 F silastic cannula (Sherwood Medical, Evry, France). Close examination of the resulting cholangiogram is essential to rule out any variations in the anatomy of the biliary tree which were not detected during probing on the backtable, such as a right branch draining into the left hepatic duct. Contrast media is rinsed out of the biliary tree with chilled UW solution.

Similarly, arteriography is done to detect arterial abnormalities, complementing the rough exploration done during backtable dissection. This precise assessment avoids an extensive dissection of the arterial tree that could jeopardize the bile duct vascularization [6, 7]. Once the anatomical reconstruction of the liver segmentation has been completely established, and therefore the level of transection of the hepatic parenchyma can be planned, the liver is returned to the ice bath of UW solution.

■ Dividing the pedicle

The inferior vena cava (IVC), median hepatic vein and the common bile duct are usually kept with the right graft. The common bile duct always stays on the right graft since variations at the confluence of the bile ducts are more common on the right than on the left, and the duct itself is usually shorter (or absent) on the right. Even more important is the arterial supply of the main bile duct being mainly derived from the right branch of the hepatic artery [8]. The left or right portal vein is cut at its origin on the portal trunk. The orifice in the portal trunk is closed with a 7/0 monofilament running suture (Teflex®, Peters, Bobigny, France). When the left branch of the portal vein is cut at its root in the portal vein, the one to three small branches arising along the first centimeter of the left branch of the portal vein are divided between ligatures. The initial mobilization permits coaxial anastomosis of the left branch of the graft's portal vein to the native portal vein, with less risk of angulation. When the artery is cut, the coeliac trunk remains with the left graft because the right branch is larger than the left one. Using an intraparenchymal suprahilar approach, the hilar plate is now brought down and the blunt metallic probe inserted into the bifurcation of the left branch to identify it. The hilar plate is cut straight with a scalpel slightly towards the left side so that the right and main hepatic ducts remain continuous. The biliary structures are thus cut blindly within the hilar plate and injury to the biliary arterial supply is minimized by less dissection.

The Spigel lobe is partially resected, ligating portal branches originating from the posterior aspect of the portal bifurcation and spigelian hepatic veins draining into the IVC. This assists implantation of the right graft in continuity with the IVC, on the native IVC when this is preserved [9].

The resection includes the *caudatus process* on the left and extends as far as the right side of the IVC. The anatomy of the termination of the main hepatic veins in the suprahepatic IVC is then inspected visually and with a probe. The end of the left hepatic vein is freed by dissection, facilitated by transection of the Arancius ligament. The main trunk is cut apart from the IVC leaving an orifice in the latter which is closed with a 4/0 running suture (Ethylon®, Ethicon, Neuilly sur Seine, France). Lengthening of the left hepatic vein stump is dangerous as it may lead to kinking of the hepatic vein anastomosis in the recipient [10].

■ Parenchymal transection

Parenchymal transection is performed straight along the middle of segment IV. Despite leaving (on both grafts) a slice of theoretically devascularized tissue during the splitting process, we have never experienced any necrosis of the cut surfaces. Depending on the desired volume of the left graft, the cutting line may be shifted to the left (when the recipients are an adult and a child, for the right and left graft, respectively), one centimeter to the right of the falciform ligament; or to the right of the middle hepatic vein, with all of segment IV being then included in the left graft (when the recipients are two adults). In the latter case, the IVC may be included in either of the grafts. When the IVC is to be resected in one of the future recipients (for example for oncological reasons), the graft to be transplanted to this recipient will retain the IVC.

A rubber tape is firmly applied to mark the proposed line of transection on the surface of the capsule of Glisson. The line is drawn from the left side of the IVC at the top, to a point equidistant from the gallbladder bed and the round ligament at the anterio-inferior limit of the liver. With the left hand acting as a block, both right and left parts tending to fall apart on each side, the liver is cut sharply with a knife along the transecting line previously marked. During this stage, a blunt metallic probe may be used to identify the position of the middle hepatic vein which is to remain on the right side. The two grafts are progressively cut apart. It is very important that the parenchyma is cut sharply in a single even plane, leaving a flat surface so that hemostatic measures may play their part most efficiently.

Using the aforedescribed procedure, as refined at our institution, the control of hemorrhage at the raw surfaces of the grafts appears to no longer be a problem [11]. This is made possible by several factors. First, the use of a scalpel to cut the liver allows one to work on a plane on which every individual cut vessel can be easily individualized and precisely closed. The cut liver offers a certain thickness which allows stitches to be

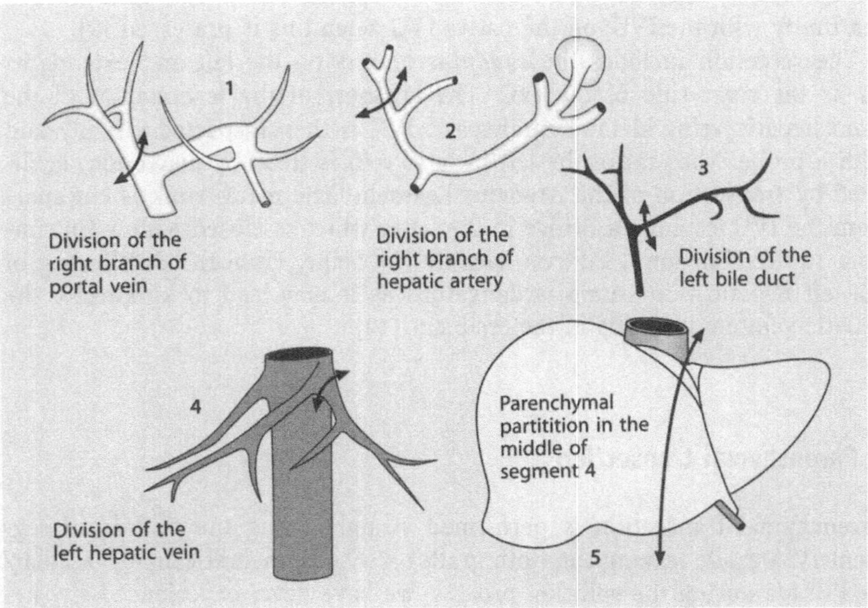

Fig. 1. Schematic representation of the basic steps of the splitting procedure. (From [11])

firmly applied. This step is time consuming and somewhat tedious. Nevertheless, in our opinion, it is a minimal price to pay considering its contribution to the effectiveness of the technique. Second, the plane surface obtained allows fibrin glue and meshes to be evenly applied.

■ Management of the cut surfaces of the grafts

First, every single vessel seen on the cut surface is closed with a 4/0 silk stitch (Peters, Bobigny, France). Running sutures may be used to close small hepatic vein branches which may have been cut longitudinally by the scalpel. Care is taken during this step to avoid liver rewarming by applying wet towels over the graft leaving only the cut surface exposed. Both surfaces of the graft are treated at the same time by two surgeons working simultaneously. When no remaining, unoccluded vessels can be seen at the liver surface, arterial, portal, biliary and hepatic venous leaks are identified for with UW injection through the corresponding hilar or caval elements. Additional stitches are applied when necessary. Second, fibrin glue is applied to the treated cut surfaces. On top of it, a hemostatic mesh (Pangen®, Laboratoires Fournier, Dijon, France) cut to the dimension of the surface is applied and sandwiched by another application of fibrin glue on top of it.

After allowing the glue to dry, a piece of resorbable mesh (Vicryl®, Ethicon, Neuilly sur Seine, France), slightly oversized as compared to the surface of the liver, is applied with glued and placed over the hemostatic mesh. The Vicryl® mesh is secured onto the liver with running sutures (Ethylon® 3/0, Ethicon, Neuilly sur Seine, France) sewing it laterally to the capsule of Glisson. The layers of mesh are cut in a customized manner at the level of the hilum so as to allow access to the elements and to avoid any compression or kinking phenomenon beneath the meshes. Interrupted stitches are used to secure the meshes at that level. Additional stitches randomly applied to the cut surfaces of the liver ensure maximal adhesion between the glued meshes and the liver surface. These stitches prevent the material from loosening and contribute to hemostasis by the compression effect the meshes exert on the cut surface. On the raw side of the graft that retains the middle hepatic vein, these stitches are put in while the vein is cannulated by the metallic probe, to avoid ligation of the vein into the graft. Each graft is weighed and any vascular modifications required are performed on the backtable. Vascular reconstructions are performed under 2.5 magnification with either 7/0 or 8/0 monofilament stitches (Teflex®, Peters, Bobigny, France).

■ Conclusion

Since the first partition of the liver was performed by Pichlmayr in 1987 [12], and one year later by Bismuth [13] refinement of the technique of split and graft implantation as described above, together with strict definition of optimal donors and grafts to be split, and a realistic selection of suitable recipients, has improved results so that morbidity, graft and patient survival are now identical using either split or whole liver for transplantation [14] with the subsequent expansion of the donor pool of organs.

■ References

1. Starzl TE, Marchioro TL, Von Kaula KN et al (1963) Homotransplantation of the liver in human. Surg. Gynecol Obstet 177:659–676
2. Azoulay D, Marin-Hargreaves G, Bismuth H (2000) Impact of liver surgery on liver transplantation. Current Opinion in Organ Transplantation 5:57–63
3. Starzl TE, Miller C, Broznick B et al (1987) An improved technique for multiple organ harvesting. Surg Gynecol Obstet 165:343–348
4. Couinaud C, Houssin D (1991) Analysis of the anatomical difficulties of bipartition. In: Couinaud C, Houssin D (eds) Controlled Partition of the Liver for Transplantation: Anatomical Limitation. Vol.1. Personal ed. Paris: Couinaud

5. Saxena R, Tokat Y, Rasmussen A et al (1995) Segmental arteries to segments I–IV from the common hepatic artery. Br J Surg 82:817–818
6. Rat P, Paris P, Friedman S et al Split-liver orthotopic liver transplantation: how to divide the portal pedicle. Surgery 1992; 112 (3):522–526
7. Cheng YF, Huang TY, Chen TY et al (1998) Radiologic anatomy in split liver transplantation. Transpl Proc 30:3184–3185
8. Stapleton GN, Hickman R, Terblanche (1998) Blood supply of the right and left hepatic ducts. Br J Surg 85:202–207
9. Lerut J, de Ville de Goyet J, Donataccio M, Reding R, Otte JB (1994) Piggyback transplantation with side-to-side cavocavostomy is an ideal technique for right split liver allograft implantation. J Am Coll Surg 179:573–576
10. Emond JC, Heffon TG, Whitington PF et al (1993) Reconstruction of the hepatic vein in reduced-size hepatic transplantation. Surg Gynecol Obst 176:11–17
11. Azoulay D, Astarcioglu I, Bismuth H et al (1996) Split-liver transplantation: the Paul Brousse policy. Ann Surg 224:737–748
12. Pichlmayr R, Ringe B, Gubernatis G et al (1988) Transplantation einer spenderleber auf zwei empfänger (splitting-transplantation): Eine neue methode in der weiterentwicklung der lebersegmenttransplantation. Langenbecks Arch Chir 373:127–130
13. Bismuth H, Morino M, Castaing D et al (1989) Emergency orthotopic liver transplantation in two patients using one donor liver. Br J Surg 76:722–724
14. Busuttil RW, Goss JA (1999) Split liver transplantation. Ann Surg 229:313–321

3.2 J. de Ville de Goyet

J. de Ville de Goyet

Technique for *ex situ* cadaveric liver graft division

■ Introduction

Although liver division for transplantation in two adults was already proposed in the past, sharing a donor liver graft has mostly concerned an adult and a child in more recent years. Interestingly, the original technique has been slightly modified with time, benefiting from technical innovations developed for procurement in living-related donors and for *in situ* division of cadaveric donor livers. These modifications for a more direct and simpler procedure.

This chapter will deal with this simpler technique which allowed safely sharing a cadaveric donor liver between a small and a larger recipient. After evaluation and simple division of the vascular structures, the liver is divided either through the umbilical scissure or along a plane left of the middle hepatic vein. Thus, the left graft consists either of segments II and III (left lateral segment graft) or segments II, III and IV, respectively. Segment IV also can be shared variably between both liver grafts (Fig. 1).

■ Definition

A "*split liver graft*" consists either of the right or left portion as obtained after division of a cadaveric donor liver graft. By definition, it implies that both halves of the donor liver are potentially functional and usable in two recipients. The key to successful liver division is to share vascular and biliary structures between the two sides but without handicapping either.

This term can also apply for a liver graft prepared strictly using the split technique, and the other liver portion discarded for logistical reasons. On the contrary, for liver grafts prepared by using similar techniques but not providing two transplantable grafts, the appellation "reduced-liver grafts" is then most appropriate.

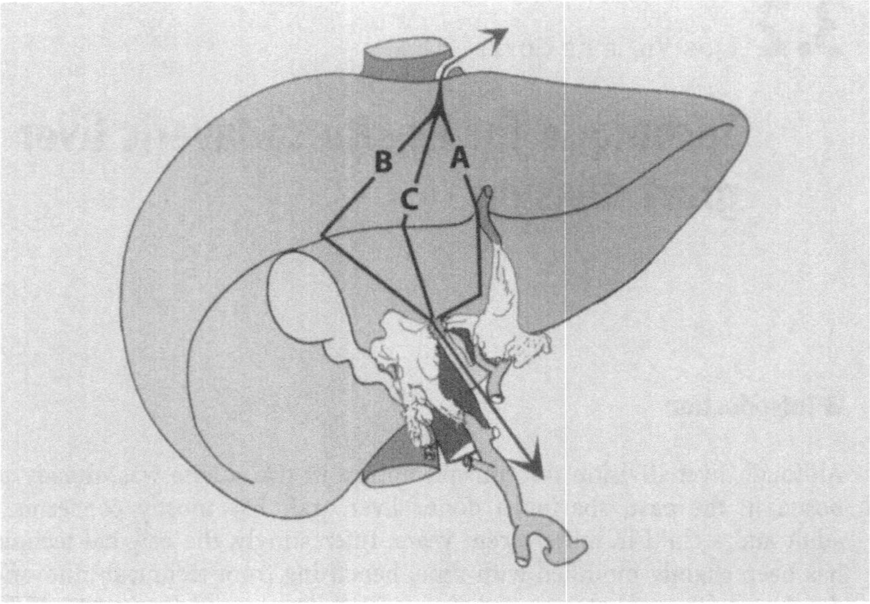

Fig. 1. Surface landmarks for liver division. The segment IV is retained with the right split graft (**a**), with the left split graft (**b**) or shared between both split grafts (**c**). Segment I is retained with the right graft

■ Donor and recipient selection

Donor selection

The benefit of split liver grafting is clearly to provide help for two recipients from one donor. Because two recipients could be put simultaneously at risk in case of liver graft primary non-function or severe dysfunction, it seems logical to avoid using livers from sub-optimal donors. Also because adding the extra backtable procedure is associated with prolongation of the ischemic time and possible related graft injury.

The following criteria can be proposed:
- donors less than 45 years old,
- hemodynamically stable (no recent severe hypotension episode or cardiac arrest),
- low or mild inotropic support,
- normal or slightly altered liver tests (less than twice the normal level),
- less than five days ITU stay,
- normal macroscopic aspect at procurement (no steatosis).

Though the latter criteria are relatively strict, at least 20–30% of the existing donor pool meet the criteria: there is thus, potentially, room for a significant increase of liver graft availability.

Recipient selection

A couple of recipients must be selected according to the donor's weight, in order to provide the necessary liver parenchymal mass to both recipients. Most often, an adult will benefit from the right graft and a child from the left graft: these grafts represent around 65% and 20–25% of the liver mass, respectively (10–15% being the estimated proportion of parenchymal loss, either segment IV or damaged parenchyma during division). In this combination, the adult recipient should be the same weight as the donor, or preferably 10 to 20% smaller, and the child weight should be 3 to 10 times less than the donor weight. These ratios would guarantee both recipients receiving at least 60% of their ideal hepatic mass, thus, avoiding the risk of severe post-transplant dysfunction. If the child weighs 3 to 4 times less than the donor, segment IV must be retained with the left graft in order to provide an adequate liver parenchymal mass to the recipient. If the ratio is more than 4, a left lateral segment split graft is appropriate (see above – Fig. 1).

Avoiding the selection of high-risk pediatric recipients for split liver graft transplantation has little sense since most urgent cases would benefit from reduced-size liver grafts, the latter sharing with split grafts similar risks related to extra backtable work and to the cut surface. On the contrary, though there is no consensus, the majority of surgeons prefer to transplant adults in elective or relatively good conditions, and avoid cases with predictable intra-operative difficulties such as known portal vein thrombosis, previous multiple operations or re-transplantation. Elective adult candidates seem to cope better with the small-for-size liver graft and the possible related functional loss, also with the possible added morbidity.

■ Procurement and logistical aspects

Conventional techniques, including "en-bloc" procedures, can be used for procurement and are not described here. Because it will be used as a separate graft, compression, excessive manipulation or trauma of the liver left lobe must be avoided during procurement. Special attention must be given to the presence of an accessory left hepatic artery, arising from the left gastric artery, which should be preserved even if small in diameter since it can represent a major vascular supply for the left lobe.

Since the main hepatic vascular structures must be shared between two grafts, surgeons must take care to provide good vascular grafts (veins and arteries) from the same donor. Long sections of the external iliac vessels provide excellent vascular allografts. Donor splenic and superior mesenteric arteries (alternatively, neck vessels) are very useful when a vascular graft is necessary for implantation of a small left or right hepatic artery.

After procurement and perfusion with preservation fluid, the liver graft is placed in sterile waterproof double bags, then in slushed ice and transported back to the transplant center. Because most cadaveric donor liver procurements are not performed at the transplant center, the transport time allows the liver graft to cool down to 0–4 °C. This is an important contribution to the prevention of ischemic injury, especially in the context of possible rewarming during backtable work. It is an important issue and the surgeon should not consider starting the liver division immediately after procuring the liver graft, but should prefer the liver resting fully immersed in ice for 1 or 2 hours before starting the backtable work.

On the other hand, efforts should be made to keep the total cold ischemic time under 12 hours when possible, again on the basis that the prolonged backtable work may allow some warming and increase the risk of preservation injury. Ideally, the liver should be stored in the ice bag for a maximum of 8 hours, less if one split liver graft must be shipped to another center after the *ex situ* procedure. Reduction of the ischemic time has been an important contributor to the improved outcome when using grafts obtained by *in situ* liver splitting (personal communications, Prof. X. Roegiers and Prof. R. Busuttil, Split Liver Symposium, March 2000, Hamburg). It thus seems logical to implement a similar approach for *ex situ* split liver graft transplantation.

■ *Ex situ* split technique

The key to successful liver division is to share vascular and biliary structures between the two sides but without handicapping either. To achieve this 'controlled liver splitting' the surgeon can follow sequential steps as suggested by Couinaud and Houssin [1–3]:

Macroscopic general evaluation of the donor liver
Conventional bench graft preparation
Evaluation of graft bilio-vascular anatomy
Liver graft division

General evaluation of the donor liver

Though the procuring surgeon already evaluated the graft quality at procurement (see above), it is good practice to re-evaluate the general liver graft and especially to avoid dividing steatotic grafts (biopsy is optional).

Because it is of importance for the post-operative hepatic function in the recipients, it is mandatory first to confirm whether both transplantations are possible, with regard to the division of parenchymal mass and respective recipient sizes. The transplant surgeon must evaluate the donor liver and the relative sizes of the right and left (possible) split grafts. This evaluation, in relation with the weight of the two potential recipients, will help confirm (or cancel) the liver graft division, also deciding whether segment IV should be kept with the right or the left graft, or shared between both grafts (Fig. 1).

This assessment also will allow the surgeon to confirm that the left split graft will fit in the recipient's abdomen, if the latter recipient is an infant and the donor is a large donor. Although successful transplantation for left lateral grafts has been reported with donor/weight ratios above 10, the use of oversized liver grafts is associated with various complications related to tight closure and graft compression with secondary ischemic damage [4–7]. The operating surgeon using visual comparison (liver segment size varies) makes a final decision regarding size match in cases with high ratios. High size mismatches is also easier accommodated when the recipient has hepatomegaly and/or ascites (up to ratio of 10), or by a technique of delayed primary closure of the abdominal wall [8] with the use of a Silastic prosthetic patch but with overlying skin closure (ratio up to 14 [9]).

Conventional bench liver graft preparation

Preparation and division of a liver requires 2 to 3 hours. Attention for maintaining adequate cooling of the graft during that period of time is essential. The following method is simple and adequate. The graft must be maintained immersed in the cold preservation fluid and shushed ice during the bench surgery, using an adequate container. The portion of the liver exposed to air can be protected by cold wet swabs regularly rinsed with the cold liquid. The conventional bench work is then done, mostly consisting of cleaning and preparing the main vascular patches and removing the gall bladder.

Evaluation of precise liver graft bilio-vascular anatomy

Hepatic arterial supply

Because the choice how to share/divide the hepatic artery between the split grafts is probably the most delicate issue, it is logical to first appreciate the precise anatomy of the arterial supply and then decide to go forward if the evaluation is favorable. The presence of accessory or variant arteries must be checked. The main hepatic artery trunk is dissected until the bifurcation into right and left branches is reached. Then the dissection is extended along the left side of the right hepatic artery in order to detect a second left hepatic artery branch: this avoids excessive freeing of the right hepatic artery from the hepatic duct (which would carry a risk of ischemic damage). Arteriography can also be useful if the arterial anatomy seems abnormal on initial inspection, thus, avoiding unnecessary extensive dissection. An on-table angiogram can be performed using contrast liquid half diluted with fresh, cold UW solution: the contrast is then flushed out by perfusing fresh UW solution.

Portal vein

The portal vein is easily dissected towards its bifurcation, using a posterior approach which best avoids dividing the important connective tissue between biliary and arterial structures. The goal of this maneuvre is to identify the portal vein bifurcation for further division. Absence of portal bifurcation (in fact absence of an extrahepatic left portal trunk) is extremely rare [1, 10, 11]: the surgeon should be aware that this would necessitate particular reconstruction, and could be considered by some workers as a contraindication for division.

Biliary tract

Dissecting bile ducts is prohibited since it would carry a risk of devascularizing the biliary tract, with subsequent ischemic damage. A cholangiography is thus performed to delineate the biliary anatomy for further division (Fig. 2). Although there is no anatomical contraindication for splitting from

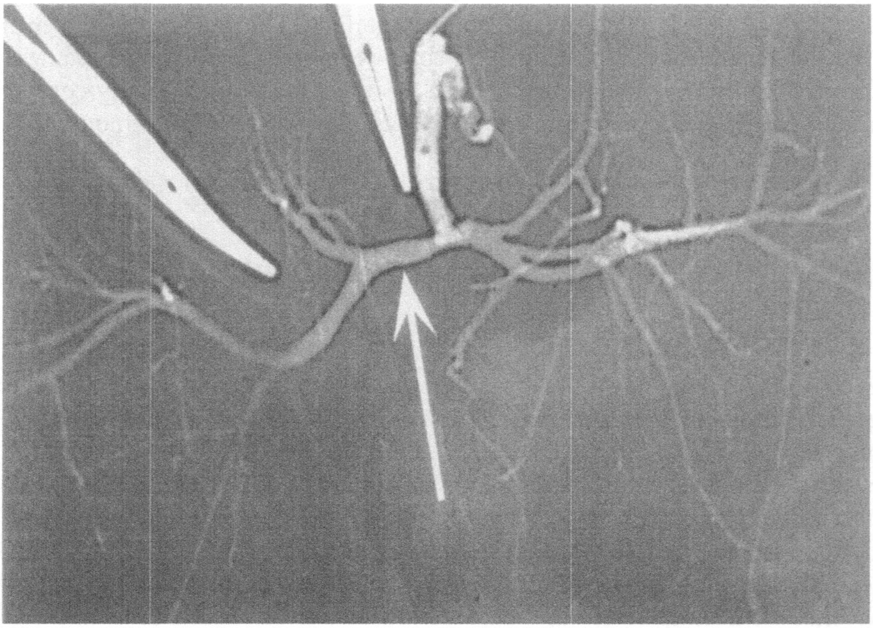

Fig. 2. Evaluation of liver graft anatomy: backtable cholangiogram. The cholangiogram is performed after positioning two clips at the porta hepatis, thus allowing precise localization of the bile duct bifurcation and of the left bile duct

a biliary tract point of view, the cholangiogram will be helpful when dividing the bilary tract. It allows avoiding trauma to the main bifurcation (which is retained with the right side) and especially in cases with a right postero-lateral duct shifted to the left (bile duct trifurcation). More importantly, it will be an important guide for dividing the left bile duct where a single trunk can be transsected (avoiding reconstruction of multiple biliary ostia; Fig. 2).

Hepatic vein

Because the *ex situ* split technique is currently used mostly for sharing a liver graft between one adult and one child, the left hepatic vein is only retained with the left graft. The vena cava and the right and middle hepatic veins are retained with the right graft. Rarely, a main left hepatic branch is found draining into the middle hepatic vein: reconstruction of this vein after division is recommended in order to avoid outflow obstruction and graft swelling. The more common variations consist of the variable length of the common middle-left hepatic venous trunk and of the presence of accessory hepatic vein collaterals (i.e., scissural or posterior branches) which do not preclude division.

Liver division

Division of the vascular structures

We share the opinion of Couinaud and Houssin [1] that division should provide both grafts with single first order arterial and biliary elements. The need for a more complex reconstruction is not a contraindication in itself but must be appropriately considered case by case, and according the team's own experience.

■ **Hepatic artery division.** The site of division of the arterial trunk is not yet standardized. Although theoretically, nearly all livers can be divided with adequate arterial reconstruction, it is recommended that each team define their own guidelines: according to their expertise, some will select only favorable conditions (a single artery for each graft) where others would accept more difficult and risky reconstructions. Also the fate of the main arterial trunk is controversial with some units preserving it preferably with the left graft and others with the right split graft. One of the arguments for keeping the main arterial trunk with the left liver is that the right artery is larger and thus less vulnerable if anastomosed directly. However microsurgical expertise, if available, should allow for many variations of arterial reconstruction, as it has been successfully implemented in living-related liver donor and *in situ* cadaveric liver graft transplantations.

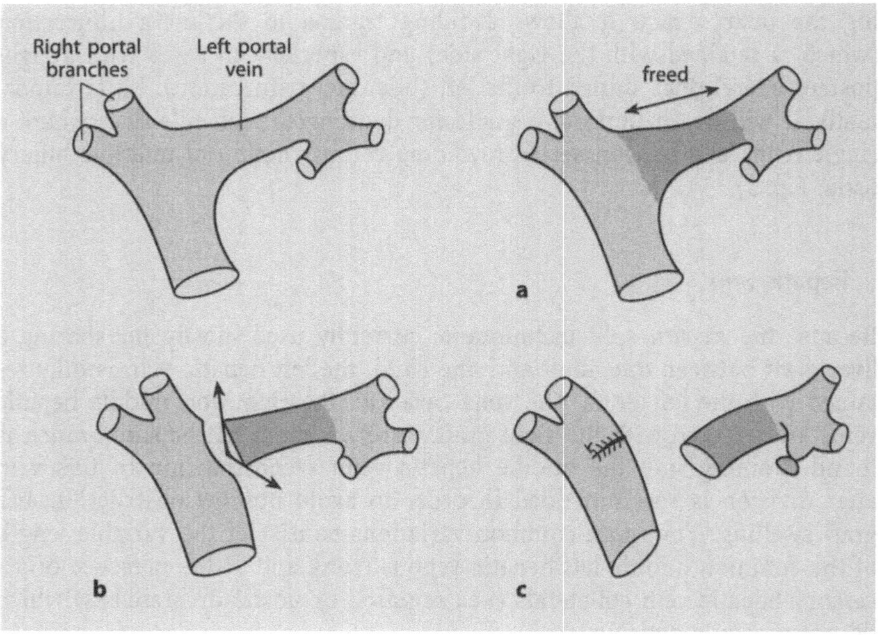

Fig. 3. Portal vein division. The left portal vein is a constant and relatively long trunk which can be kept for the left graft after mobilization (**a**). The vein is divided flush from the portal trunk which is reconstructed by transverse suturing

■ **Portal vein division.** Many surgeons prefer to keep the main portal vein with the right liver [12–15]. This is easily done when the left portal trunk has been freed from its attachement to the hilar plate (which implies dividing branches towards segment I). The 2–3 cm vein length thereby provided facilitates subsequent anastomosis to the recipient portal vein or to a vein graft (if additional length is necessary) (Fig. 3).

■ **Biliary tract division.** The cholangiogram (see above) is helpful to guide the surgeon: the ideal site for division is located at some distance from the main bile duct confluence, while providing a single left bile duct with the left split graft (Fig. 2).

■ **Hepatic vein.** The left hepatic vein is divided at its ostium, thus retaining a small venous cuff: the latter cuff is a patch taken from the portion of the vena cava immediately above and behind the former ostium. The residual defect is closed preferably by a direct transverse suturing or using a venous patch (donor allograft) (Fig. 4). Rarely, a large venous branch from segment III drains into the middle hepatic vein at some distance from the ostium: this branch is then divided during the parenchymal transection and

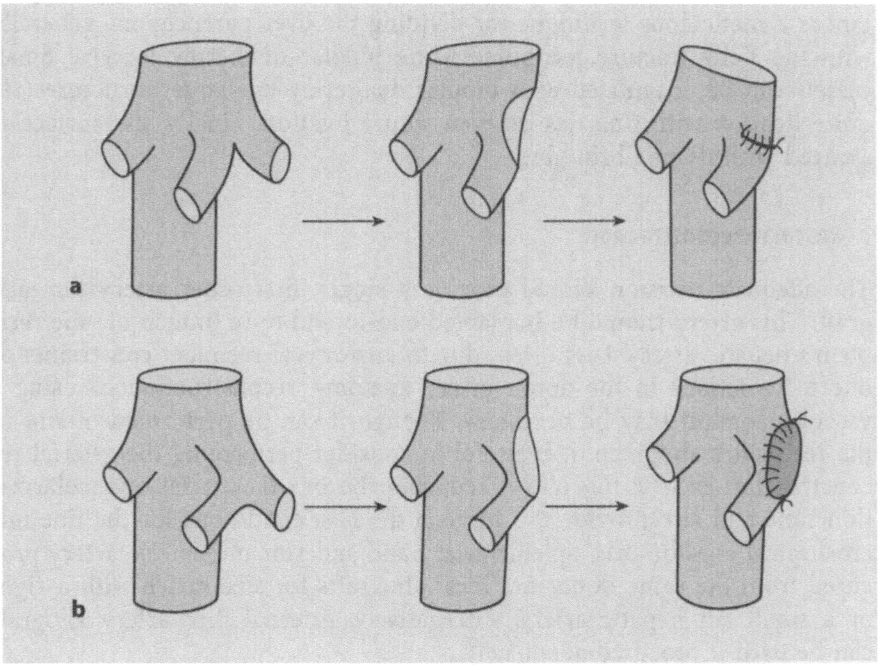

Fig. 4. Hepatic vein division. The left hepatic vein is divided by retaining a short patch from the vena cava (**a**). The defect is then easily closed by transverse suturing. When middle and left hepatic veins share a long common trunk, a small venous patch (donor vascular graft) is best appropriate (**b**)

graft swelling could occur if it is tied off. Alternatively, a jump venous allograft reconstruction onto the vena cava can be considered.

Parenchymal section/cut surface hemostasis

Most often the division line follows the falciform ligament providing a small left split graft for a small recipient. A variation consists of retaining a variable portion of the segment IV (Fig. 1) which allows transplanting the left graft into slightly larger pediatric recipients. The section plane is then shifted towards the middle hepatic vein, retaining the latter vein with the right graft. The caudate lobe (segment I) is usually kept with the right side, or alternatively can be resected (this maneuvre facilitates further cavo-cavostomy if the latter is the surgeon's choice).

Though persisting controversy regarding that segment IV would become necrotic if retained with the right graft, in practice this has not been found to be of clinical significance. Moreover, retention of segment IV with the right side reduces the cut surface area and may reduce bleeding. Alternatively, some prefer discarding segment IV when it is not retained with the left split graft.

Hemostasis of the cut surface is achieved by various means. Most important is a meticulous technique for dividing the liver parenchyma, generally with the Kelly fracture technique using bipolar diathermy forceps. Small vessels can be coagulated with bipolar diathermy but larger structures require ligation with fine ties or even suture ligation. Finally, the surface is sprayed with tissue fibrin glue.

Vascular reconstruction

The adequate division should provide a single, first order artery for each graft. This artery should be implanted end-to-end to (a branch of) the recipient's hepatic artery. Less often, due to anatomical recipient constraints or due to variations in the donor artery anatomy, reconstruction or using a vascular conduit may be necessary. Though it can be performed *in situ* in the recipient's abdomen, it is useful to consider performing the arterial reconstruction *ex situ*: this allows reducing the *in situ* arterial revascularization time and also provide the surgeon the best conditions for the fine microsurgical anastomosis. Splenic artery and superior mesenteric artery procured from the same donor are ideal allografts for size-match with a right or a small left hepatic artery. Alternatively, external iliac artery allograft can be used if procured adequately.

As in conventional transplantation, some recipient anatomical particularities may need interposing a donor vascular graft (i.e., portal vein thrombosis or hypoplasia, need for jump graft to aorta) which is done using well-known techniques.

As described above, a venous patch vena cava repair can be useful after hepatic vein divison, and a jump graft interposition is rarely necessary.

■ Transplantation of split liver grafts

As obtained using the above described technique (Figs. 1 and 5), the right and left split grafts are easily implanted using well-described conventional techniques for orthotopic full size or left lateral segment transplantation. The main variation resides in the short hepatic vein cuff provided with the left split graft: this is usually easily overcome by using the triangular piggy-back anastomosing technique onto the recipient hepatic vein ostia [16].

■ Comments

Although the first cases were reported as early as 1988 [17, 18], only 100 split liver graft transplantations were reported 4 years later, in 1993, at the first symposium dedicated to this technique [13]. Another 200 were per-

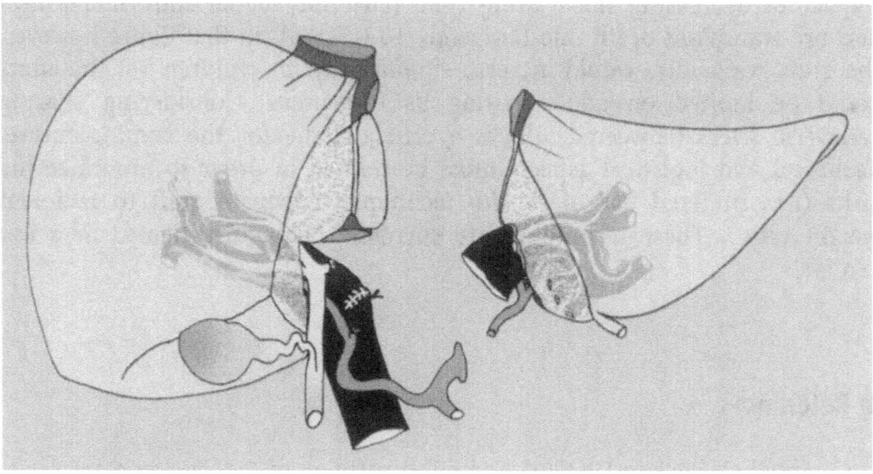

Fig. 5. Right and left split graft: final aspect. In this standard preparation, the left graft (segments II and III) is procured with the left portal vein, the left hepatic artery and the left bile duct. The portal trunk, celiac axis and common bile duct are retained with right split graft (segments I, IV, V, VI, VII, VIII)

formed within the next 3 years and a total of 300 split liver grafts were reported at the second symposium in 1996 (unpublished data). Although this showed a slight trend for increased use, these numbers did not compare favorably with the contemporary rates of conventional transplants in Europe (around 2500 per year) and with the rapid expansion of living-related donor programs worldwide (around 200 per year after 1995).

Skepticism and continuing debates regarding the real benefit of implementing these techniques in routine was initially based on some less than satisfactory results reported in the very early experience. This opinion persisted until the late 1990s despite a clear correlation being established between the poor results and the selection of high-risk candidates, the excessively long ischemic times, or the use of sub-optimal donors. However, several centers cautiously pursued developing split programs. Larger single-center series are now available in the literature [19–23] and their results confirm that an excellent outcome can be achieved.

In the context of persisting organ shortage and death of candidates while waiting for a graft, the increasing competition for healthy adult livers between pediatric and adult recipients makes it necessary to abandon the reduction techniques (which discard the right lobe), when possible, and favor splitting the liver graft for two recipients. Selecting adequate donors, graft with favorable anatomy and stable recipients seems important, at least during the learning curve.

As proposed by Busuttil et al. [24] in a recent review paper, national liver graft allocation organizations should consider "intend to split policy" in the future. There is little doubt that a split policy would have a strong impact in decreasing the waiting time (currently persistently increasing) and pre-transplant death rate (currently 10 to 15%). In that figure however, the graft availability would increase significantly for children but the effect could be limited on adult waiting list dynamics. Considering sharing cadaveric livers between adults is a critical issue for the coming future. Technical and logistical aspects must be refined in order to minimize the risks (i.e., prefered use of *in situ* technique, adequate graft to recipient weight ratio). These techniques are currently being investigated in a few centers.

References

1. Couinaud C, Houssin D (1991) Controlled partition of the liver for transplantation. Anatomical limitations. In: Personal Edition (eds) Paris, pp 1–80
2. Couinaud C, Houssin D (1992) Bipartage réglé en vue de transplantation. Simplification de la méthode. Chirurgie 118:217–222
3. Houssin D, Boillot O, Soubrane O, Couinaud C, Pitre J, Ozier Y, Devictor D, Bernard O, Chapuis Y (1993) Controlled liver splitting for transplantation in two recipients: technique, results and perspectives. Br J Surg 80:75–80
4. de Hemptinne B, de Ville de Goyet J, Kestens PJ, Otte JB (1987) Volume reduction of the liver graft before orthotopic transplantation: report of a clinical experience in 11 cases. Transplant Proc 19:3317–3322
5. Ong TH, Lynch SV, Pillay SP, Balderson GA, Wall DR, Shepherd R, Cleghorn G, Patrick M, De Buse P, Clark R, Board AJ, Lister B, Kato K, Hardie IR, Strong RW (1989) Reduced-size orthotopic liver transplantation in children: an experience with seven cases. Transplant Proc 21:2443–2444
6. Badger IL, Czerniak A, Beath S, Tisone G, Deakin M, Sherlock DJ, Kelly DA, Mc Master P, Buckels JAC (1992) Hepatic transplantation in children using reduced size allograft. Br J Surg 79:47–49
7. Soubrane O, Dousset B, Ozier Y, Devictor D, Pariente D, Bernard O, Houssin D, Chapuis Y (1990) The choice of the reduction technique for orthotopic liver transplantation (OLT) in children using a reduced-size graft. Transplant Proc 22: 1147–1148
8. de Ville de Goyet J, Struye de Swielande Y, Reding R, Sokal E, Otte JB (1998) Delayed primary closure of the abdominal wall after cadaveric and living related donor liver graft transplantation in children: a safe and useful technique. Transpl Int 11:117–122
9. de Ville de Goyet J, Reding R, Lerut J, Sokal E, Otte JB (1999) Paediatric orthotopic liver transplantation: lessons from a single center experience with 532 transplants in 446 children. Acta Gastro-enterol Belg 62:290–294
10. Atri M, Bret PM, Fraser-Hill MA (1992) Intrahepatic portal venous variations: prevalence with US. Radiology 184:157–158
11. Hardy KJ, Nye DH (1969) An abnormal portal vein. pp 676–681
12. de Ville de Goyet J, Otte JB (1995) Cut-Down and Split liver transplantation. In: Philadelphia Saunders, pp 481–496
13. de Ville de Goyet J (1995) Split liver transplantation in Europe, 1988 to 1993. Transplantation 59:1371–1376

14. Otte JB, de Ville de Goyet J, Alberti D, Balladur P, de Hemptinne B (1990) The concept and technique of the split liver in clinical liver transplantation. Surgery 107:605–612
15. Rat P, Paris P, Friedman S, Favre JP (1992) Split-liver orthotopic liver transplantation: how to divide the portal pedicle. Surgery 112:522–526
16. Emond JC, Heffron TG, Whitington PF, Broelsch CE (1993) Reconstruction of the hepatic vein in reduced size hepatic transplantation. Surg Gynecol Obstet 176:11–17
17. Bismuth H, Morino M, Castaing D, Gillon MC, Descorps-Declere A, Saliba F, Samuel D (1989) Emergency orthotopic liver transplantation in two patients using one donor liver. Br J Surg 76:722–724
18. Pichlmayr R, Ringe B, Gubernatis G, Hauss J, Bunzendahl H (1988) Transplantation einer Spenderleber auf zwei Empfänger (splitting- transplantation) - Eine neue Methode in der Weiterentwicklung der Lebersegmenttransplantation. Langenbecks Arch Chir 373:127–130
19. Mirza D, Achilleos OA, Pirenne J, Buckels JAC, McMaster P, Mayer AD (1998) Encouraging results of split-liver transplantation. Br J Surg 85:494–497
20. Rela M, Vougas V, Muisan P, Vilca-Melandez H, Smyrmiotis V, Gibbs P, Karani J, Williams R, Heaton N (1998) Split liver transplantation. Ann Surg 227:282–288
21. Azoulay D, Astarologlu I, Bismuth H, Castaing D, Majno P, Adam R, Johann M (1996) Split-liver transplantation. The Paul-Brousse policy. Ann Surg 224:737–748
22. Rogiers X, Malago M, Gawad K, Kuhlencordt R, Fröschle G, Sturm E, Sterneck M, Pothmann W, Schulte Am Esch J, Burdelski M, Broelsch CE (1996) One year experience with extended application and modified techniques of split liver transplantation. Transplantation 61:1059–1061
23. Kalayoglu M, D'Alessandro AM, Knechtle SJ, Hoffmann RM, Pirsch JD, Judd RH, Armbrust M, Spaith E, Pilli G, Young CJ, Geffner SR, Odorico JS, Sollinger HW, Belzer FO (1996) Preliminary experience with split liver transplantation. J Am Coll Surg 182:381–387
24. Busuttil RW, Goss JA (1999) Split liver transplantation. Ann Surg 229:313–321

3.3 Technique of left lateral *in situ* splitting

D.C. Broering, C. Hillert, and X. Rogiers

Introduction

Split liver transplantation (SLT) has emerged to a standard procedure in liver transplantation during the last 10 years. The procedure is the logical consequence in the technical development of liver transplantation.

The technique of harvesting the left lateral liver lobe from a living donor inspired Rogiers et al. to develop the *in situ* split technique, which was first performed in our center in 1995 [1]. Split liver transplantation provides an ideal means of generating size-matched liver grafts for children without reducing the organ pool for adult recipients. Today, *in situ* split liver transplantation is an established procedure with excellent and comparable results to *ex situ* splitting and whole liver transplantation. The procurement of the left lateral liver lobe (segments II, III) is performed in the heart-beating cadaveric donor with standard surgical facilities for a multiorgan harvesting.

We describe the standardized technique of left lateral in situ splitting used in the Department for Hepatobiliary Surgery at the University Hospital Eppendorf in Hamburg.

Exploration – anatomy – graft quality

The abdomen is opened through a midline laparotomy and sternotomy. After opening, a thorough exploration of the abdominal cavity and the vascular anatomy and quality of the liver is performed. Only hemodynamically stable cadaveric donors with good liver quality (fatty degeneration less than 30%) are eligible for *in situ* splitting. The age of the donor should be less than 50 years and stay on ICU less than 5 days. Only the visual assessment of an experienced split liver transplant surgeon usually decides if the liver is splitable.

Anatomical variations of the liver's vascular supply are technical challenges, which might obviate liver splitting. In general the left liver carries fewer anatomical variants than the right liver. Especially the left lateral lobe has shown to be very constant regarding anatomy. Contraindications for a left lateral splitting are the absence of the left portal vein or left main bile duct. Severe malformations of the arterial trunk to the left lateral graft can also serve as contraindications for splitting. Intraoperative ultrasound, if available in the donor hospital, of the donor liver can help to evaluate venouse anatomy of the left lateral lobe.

■ Mobilization of the left lateral liver lobe

An abdominal pad is placed behind the segments II and III to allow safe transsection of the left triangular ligament with electrocautery (Fig. 1). The attachments to the diaphragm are cut in the same manner. The left hepatic lobe is lifted with a retractor and the lesser omentum, is dissected. During dissection of the lesser omentum, care has to be taken to identify a replaced hepatic artery.

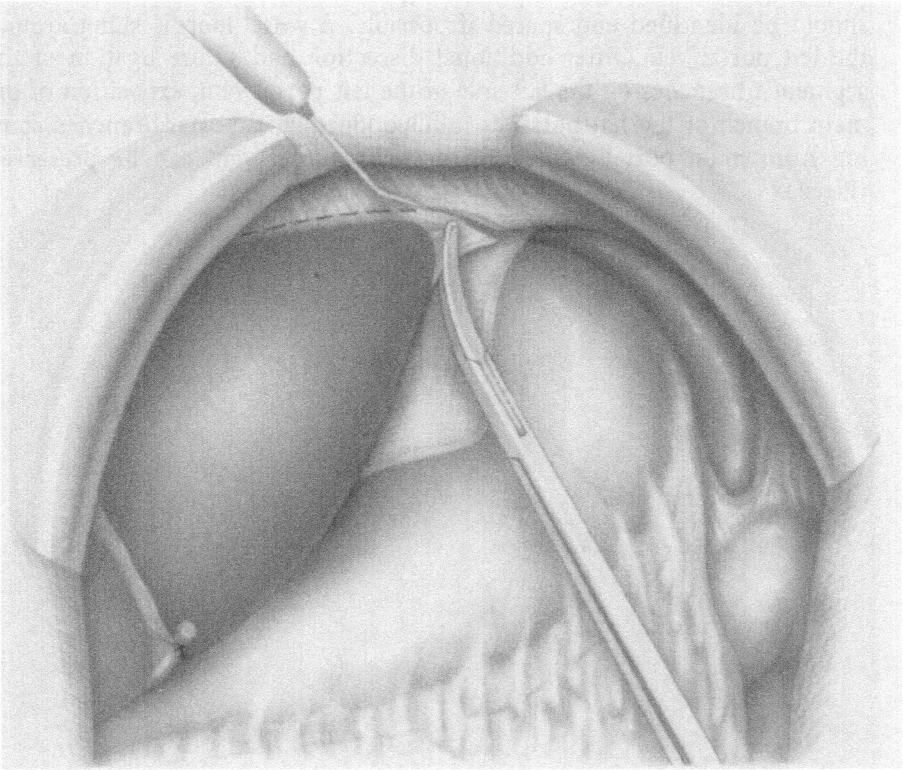

Fig. 1. Mobilization of the left lateral liver lobe. Transsection of the left triangular ligament by electrocautery

■ Dissection of the left hepatic artery and left portal vein

The anterior peritoneal sheath of the left part of the hepatoduodenal ligament is opened. The level of dissection is defined by the lower margin of segment IV and the left hepatic artery (Fig. 2). The left hepatic artery is dissected throughout its length until its course to the left liver can safely be identified and is marked with a vessel loop. During this step, dissection has to be performed with caution to avoid any trauma with following intimal dissection and thrombosis of the left hepatic artery. If a segment IV artery, arises from left hepatic artery or propria hepatic artery, it should also be dissected until its course to segment IV. Dissection of the right hepatic artery and propria hepatic artery is unnecessary and increase only the risk of arterial complications to the right extended graft.

In the following step the parenchymal bridge between segment IV and III is transected by electrocautery. Sometimes, however, sutures may be necessary to achieve complete bilio- and hemostasis. Then the ligamentum teres hepatis is separated from peritoneal adhesions towards the quadrate lobe. The peritoneal sheath is opened on the right side of the umbilical recessus. The delicate portal branches towards segment IV are prepared and suture-ligated with 5-0 sutures. During these steps the segment IV artery should be identified and spared if possible. A vessel-loop is slung around the left portal vein. After additional dissection and suture ligation of the segment I branches on the left side of the left portal vein, exposition of the main branch of the left portal is fulfilled. Segment I portal branches coming from main portal bifurcation or main portal vein can be preserved (Fig. 3).

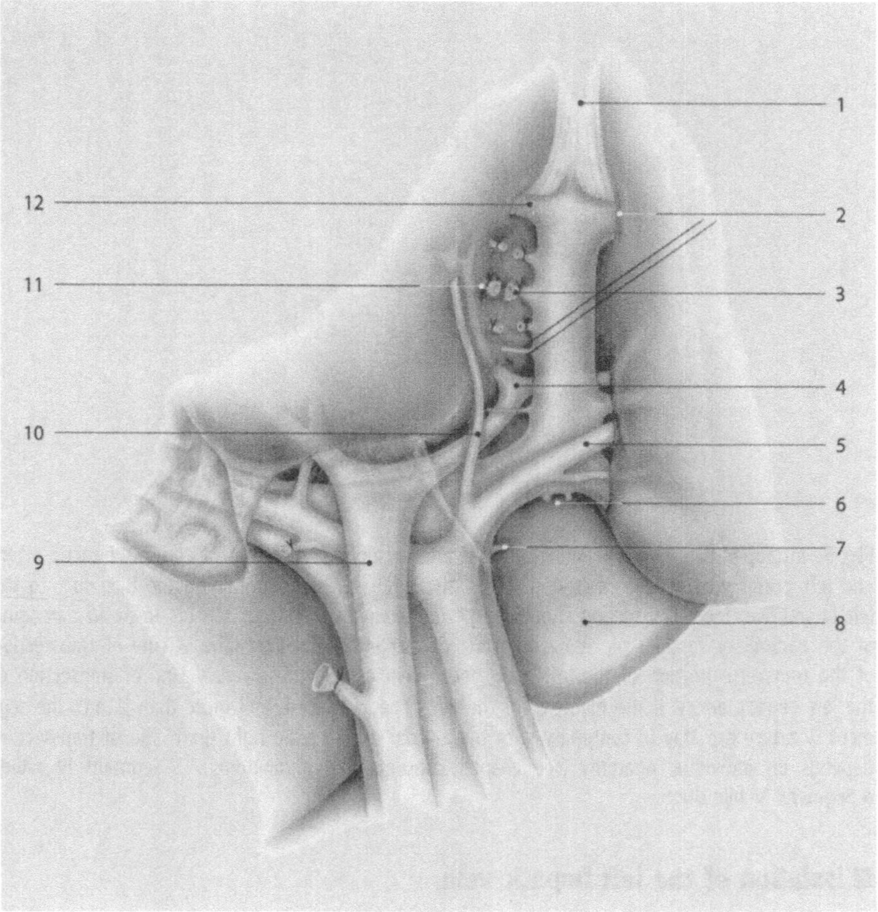

Fig. 2. Situation after dissection of the left hepatic artery and identification of segment IV artery. The peritoneum at the right border of the umbilical portion of the left portal vein is opened after transection of the small parenchymal bridge between lobus quadratus and segment III to gain excess to the portal segment IV branches. Note, that the peritoneal sheet covering the main hepatoduodenal ligament and the right extremity of the this ligament remains untouched to prevent any damage to the bile duct and vascular structues of the right extended lobe. *1* Umbilical ligament. *2* Large portal branch to segment III from umbilical portion of the left portal vein. *3* Stump of segment IV portal vein branch after ligation. Note that only selective suture ligation of this branch is allowed to prevent closure of adjacent segment IV artery and bile duct. *4* Union of segment IV bile duct and bile duct from left lateral lobe at the right extremity of the umbilical portion of the left portal vein. *5* Left hepatic artery. *6* Portal segment I branches which have to be transected. *7* Portal vein branch to segment I which can be preserved to achieve portal inflow to segment I. *8* Caudate lobe (segment I). *9* Common hepatic duct. *10* Segment IV artery arising from the left hepatic artery. *11* Segment IV bile duct. *12* Large segment IV portal branch, which has to be transected to achieve access behind the umbilical portion ofthe left portal vein and the umbilical plate

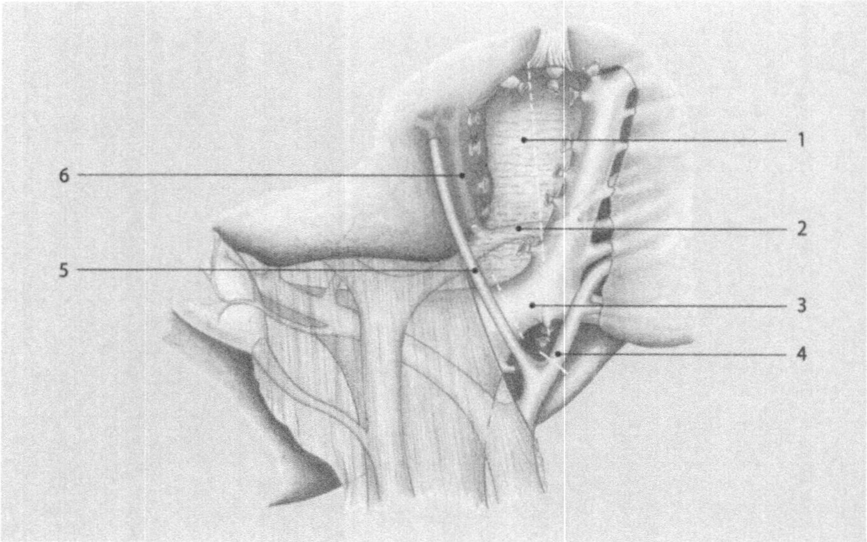

Fig. 3. Intraoperative view on umbilical plate after complete dissection of the left hepatic artery and left portal vein. *1* Line of transection of the umbilical plate containing the bile duct to the left lateral liver lobe. Transection should be performed with a knife or scissors to avoid damaging of the parabiliary vascular plexus. *2* Bile duct of the left lateral liver lobe. *3* Line of transsection of the transverse portion of the left main portal vein can be preserved. *4* Line of transection of the left hepatic artery. If the diameter of the left hepatic artery is still more than 2 mm, the segment IV artery can stay in continuity with the arterial trunk to the right graft. Site of transsection depends on individual anatomy (see chapter consequences of anatomy). *5* Segment IV artery. *6* Segment IV bile duct

■ Isolation of the left hepatic vein

The obliterated ductus venosum within the sulcus of arantius has to be dissected until its course into the vena cava. The fibrotic remnant of ductus venosum can be used to expose the space between the vena cava and the left hepatic vein while pulling it to the left. Then the left hepatic vein is cautiously dissected ventrocranially and dorsocaudally using an Overholt clamp (Fig. 4). This step should only be performed if it is easily feasible. Any hazard or forced steps should be avoided to beware damaging or opening of a large vein. After isolation of the left hepatic vein is accomplished, dissection of the liver parenchyma can be started.

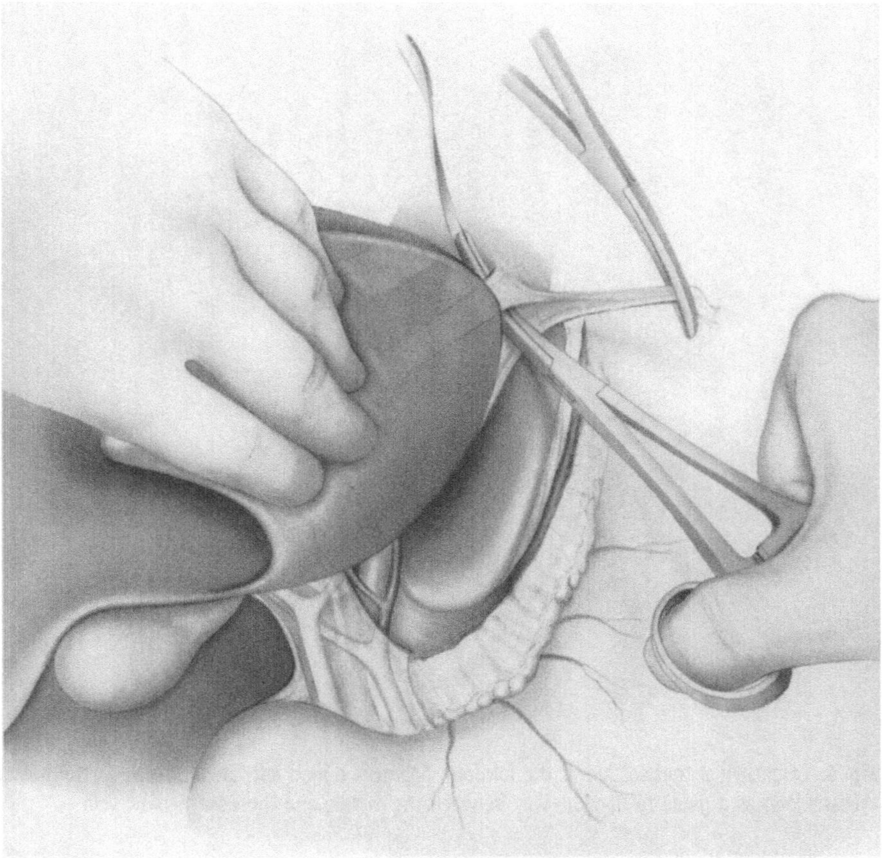

Fig. 4. Technique of safe isolation of the left hepatic vein

■ Dissection of the parenchyma and division of the umbilical plate

The liver capsule is marked with electrocautery. The plane of parenchymal division is defined by the falciform ligament. Since there are only a few vessels in this layer between segments II and IV, bleeding is limited. The dissection of the liver parenchyma is performed in small steps using the Harmonic Scapel (Ethicon, Nordersted, Germany) or an ultrasound dissector (CUSA). Parenchymal transsection with electocautery or finger fracture should be avoided to minimize the risk of major bleeding and narrowing the middle or left hepatic vein during the last phase of transsection.

The parenchyma is dissected down to the umbilical plate. The umbilical plate, containing the left lateral bile duct is controlled with a right angled clamp passing behind the umbilical plate. Transsection of the umbilical plate is performed using a scalpel or vascular scissors. Any kind of electrocautery in this region has to be avoided to protect the left lateral bile duct

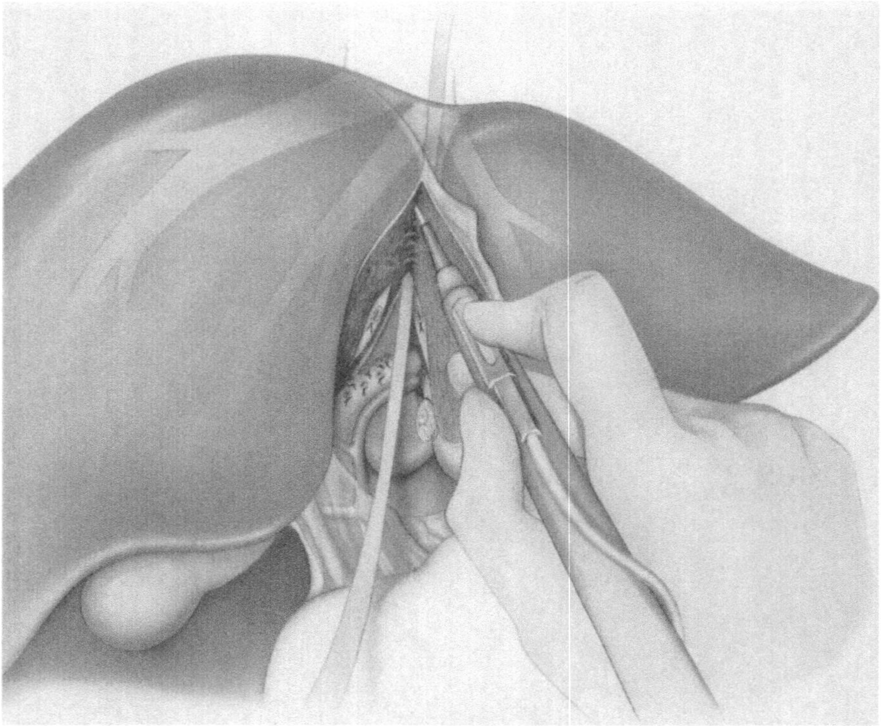

Fig. 5. Parenchymal transsection at the falciform ligament during left lateral *in situ* splitting using a vessel-loop as a guide to find the way between the middle and the right hepatic vein

from devascularization. Arterial bleeding from the left stump of the umbilical plate should controlled only by compression. Stitching of these small arterial bleedings carries the risk of closing significant adjacent bile ducts of the left lateral lobe. On the right side oversewing of the stump of the left bile duct is performed using resorbable suture material. During this step complete oversewing of the stump of the umbilical plate with a running suture is crucial to close any additional tiny bile ducts, which otherwise lead to bile leakage.

Now the left end of the vessel-loop, slung around the left hepatic vein, is passed behind the left lateral lobe and anterior to the left portal vein and left hepatic artery. After this maneuver the vessel-loop serves as a guide to maintain the right direction during transsection of the liver between the left and middle hepatic veins [2] (Fig. 5).

Small vein branches are isolated and suture ligated or clipped. Once the last part of the parenchyma is cut the vessel-loop comes free and division of the liver is accomplished. Throughout the entire preparation the right part of the hepatoduodenal ligament has remained untouched.

■ Explantation

Now the donor has two livers, which can be perfused before procurement. Both grafts can be perfused and removed together as in a routine procurement [3]. Alternatively harvesting and backtable perfusion of the left lateral graft can be performed as applied in living donation if logistical reasons emphasize this. For this the left hepatic artery is clamped at it origin from the propria hepatic artery and cut. The left portal vein is cut at the transverse portion of the left portal vein. Once the left hepatic vein is clamped and transected, the left lateral graft is transferred to the backtable and flushed with preservation solution. The vascular stumps of the right liver are sutured. For safety reasons the venous stump is sutured twice. The stump of the portal vein has to be closed in a transverse manner to avoid any narrowing of the main portal vein bifurcation. Arteries are sutured-ligated. Using this technique there is no need for compressing mattress sutures. Before explantation of the right lobe, perfusion of segment I and IV can be observed.

■ Conclusion

In situ left lateral split liver transplantation has been proven to be a successful and reliable procedure in liver transplantation. The procedure has shown to be teachable and applicable also in small donor hospitals, thus, only increasing the time for organ procurement to 1 hour. There are fewer biliary complications with *in situ* splitting, which may be explained by the greater amount of anatomical dissection with this technique. The perfect hemostasis at the time of reperfusion offers a better overview of the situation for the implant surgeon. But the main advantage of *in situ* splitting is to avoid prolonging the ischemic time, which is still an important risk factor in liver transplantation.

■ References

1. Rogiers X, Malago M, Gawad K, Jauch KW, Olausson M, Knoefel WT, Gundlach M, Bassas A, Fischer L, Sterneck M, Burdelski M, Broelsch CE (1996) In situ splitting of cadaveric livers. The ultimate expansion of a limited donor pool. Ann Surg 224:331–339
2. Broering DC, Rogiers X, Malago M, Bassas A, Broelsch CE (1998) Vessel loop-guided technique for parenchymal transection in living donor or in situ split-liver procurement. Liver Transpl Surg 4(3):241
3. Busuttil RW, Goss JA (1999) Split liver transplantation. Ann Surg 229(3):313–321

3.4

J. Belghiti, G.M Ettore, D. Sommacale, A. Sauvanet, and O. Farges

In situ splitting "full right – full left" for two adult recipients

Introduction

Ex situ split liver transplantation from cadaveric donors is an attractive concept allowing transplantation of two recipients with a single liver [1]. However, this technique did not gain wide acceptance because it was associated with increased morbidity and reduced graft survival [2]. The main drawbacks were a risk of bleeding from the cut surface, a high incidence of biliary complications and a prolonged cold ischemia time [2]. To overcome these problems, Rogiers et al. described an *in situ* splitting procedure which was associated with reduced cold ischemia time, incidence of biliary complications and primary delayed function as well as with improved graft and patient survival rates compared with the *ex situ* splitting [3]. However, whether performed *ex situ* or *in situ*, splitting techniques generate left grafts of limited size as it is usually agreed that the middle hepatic vein belongs to the right liver [4]. Transection is therefore either performed at the level of the falciform ligament [5, 6] or in the middle of segment IV [7] but with the middle hepatic vein being retained with the right graft. With these techniques, it has very seldom been possible to obtain a left graft large enough for an adult recipient.

We herein describe a modification of the *in situ* splitting technique consisting in a transection performed along the main portal fissure retaining the middle hepatic vein with the left graft. This modification generated two grafts of comparable size allowing the safe transplantation of two adult recipients.

Selection of donor

All of our cases of *in situ* "full right – full left" splitting were considered in adults aged less than 50 years weighting more than 75 kg, excluding patients with chronic alcohol consuption and/or GGT > 2 N. Only hemodynamically stable cadaveric donors were selected. Using these criteria we do not exclude patients with renal or pulmonary failure including those with duration of ICU stay prior to organ harvesting >5 days. All of the donors were harvested at our institution; in the first case we performed angiography showing a normal arterial and portal supply to the liver and computed tomography in order to evaluate the volume of the left liver (segments II, III and IV). With greater experience we exclusively used the US evaluation with a special reference to the presence of steatosis and the portal distribution. We excluded patients with dysmorphic liver and patients in whom the right anterior sector is drained into the left portal branch. Our two first cases were not a part of a multiorgan procurement. In cases of multiorgan procurement, the cardiothoracic surgeon was asked to come 2 hours later than usual.

■ Recipient selection

Transplantations with the right and left grafts were performed in our institution in low-risk patients (UNOS 3 & 4), matched during the weekly transplant conference. The selection of the patients allocated to the right graft is very large, excluding patients weighting more than 100 kg and those who underwent a previous liver surgical procedure allowing us to foresee technical difficulties. On the other hand, the selection of the adult patient allocated to the left graft was very limited, selecting patients weighting less than 55 kg without a previous abdominal procedure. Our goal is to provide a graft volume of 1% of the body weight of the recipient.

■ Donor procedure

The liver procurement team included one senior surgeon with experience in living-donor liver procurement. The infrarenal aorta and vena cava were dissected free and controlled so that rapid perfusion was possible in case of donor instability. After inspection of the liver, evaluating the size of both right and left livers, intraoperative US was used in all cases assessing the vascular anatomy with special attention to the anatomy of the hepatic veins. Cholecystectomy was performed and the cystic duct was cannulated for intraoperative cholangiography. When a normal biliary distribution was assessed, the two recipients are transported to the operating room. The cannula was also used after liver transection for detecting bile leakage by injection of methylene blue into the common bile duct. After mobilization of the left lateral lobe (segments II and III), the common trunk of the middle and left hepatic veins was controlled extraparenchymally as well as the origin of the right and left branches of the common hepatic artery and portal vein. Parenchymal transection was performed using an ultrasonic dissector (Dissectron, Satelec Medical, Mérignac, France) and bipolar electric cautery along the main portal fissure without clamping and with minimal manipulation. The hepatic veins of segments V and VIII were divided close to their termination in the middle hepatic vein, but the main trunk of the middle hepatic vein was retained with the left graft. The left biliary duct was cut in the hilar plate without attempting to encircle it. When the section plane overtakes the plane of the middle hepatic vein, we move to a horizontal plane along a course from the Cantlie's line to the Arantius' ligament. After total parenchymal division, the ideal situation is to maintain *in situ* perfusion of the split liver until the two hepatectomies had been completed in order to minimize cold ischemia time. Then the left hepatic graft was removed with division of the afferent and efferent vessels at their origin. The left graft was delivered into a basin containing ice slush and infused with 1000 mL UW solution through the portal vein. When the orifice of the middle and left hepatic vein are separated, a common anastomotic orifice is reconstructed and the left graft can be immediatly transplanted to the first recipient with an ischemic duration as short as possible.

The right graft (comprising segments V to IX and I and the retrohepatic IVC) was not mobilized during the whole procedure. The vascular and biliary branches of the remaining liver were suture ligated and hemostasis of the cut surface was completed, taking advantage of the preservation of both portal and arterial perfusion and of the donor's intact coagulation. However, at this step the *in situ* procedure can be interrupted without any deleterious consequence, the further procurement being like that of routine multiorgan – donor procedure.

■ Recipients procedure

Surgery in both recipients was initiated simultaneously and immediately after the cholangiography in the donor had confirmed that splitting was possible. Both patients underwent total hepatectomy with preservation of the portal and caval flows. The left graft can be immediately transplanted while less than 30 minutes of backtable preparation of the IVC is required before implantation of the right graft. In both recipients, vascular reconstruction can be performed without graft interposition. Biliary reconstruction is performed by a Roux en Y anastomosis in the recipient of the left graft and by bilio-biliary anastomosis in the recipient of the right graft.

■ Results and discussion

Initial reports of right liver procurement either by *ex vivo* or *in situ* splitting were all described with the middle hepatic vein being retained with the right graft [3, 5–10] because it was feared that congestion would other-

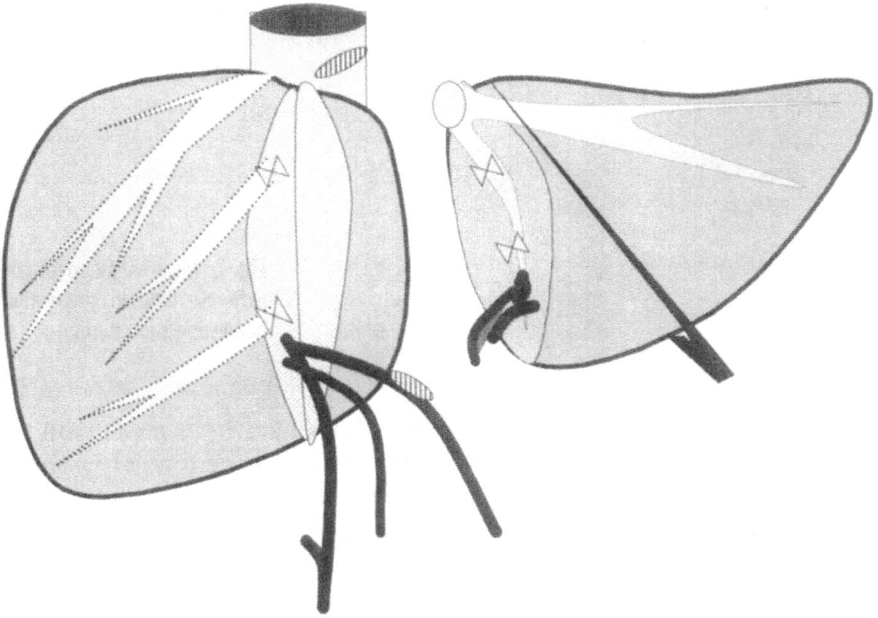

Fig. 1. Diagrammatic representation of the anatomy of the two grafts

wise occur. This assumption was based on anatomical works showing that the middle hepatic vein predominantly drains the right liver and in particular segments V and VIII, which have a separate drainage in this vein (Fig. 1). However, this assumption is not supported during living-related transplantation when the full left liver comprising segments II to IV with the middle and left hepatic veins was harvested without any obvious congestion in the remnant right liver. Similarly living-related transplantations of right livers comprising segments V to VIII only drained by the right hepatic vein can be successfully performed with the middle hepatic vein being preserved in the donor [11]. A possible interpretation of this apparent discrepancy between anatomical works and clinical experience is that an effective venous collateral circulation develops during *in vivo* liver transection, especially when it is performed without clamping of the hepatic pedicle, whereas it may not develop when transection is performed *ex situ*. In case of large veins draining segments V and/or VIII to the middle hepatic vein, we believe that the IVC should be harvested with this part of the liver, to allow an easy and large cavocaval anastomosis and to preserve the inferior and accessory hepatic veins that contribute to the venous drainage of the right liver through the dorsal sector. This technique may allow better venous drainage than that reported by Colledan et al. [12] who suggested retaining the donor's IVC with the left graft. For the left graft, we have found that the common trunk of the left and middle hepatic veins allowed a wide anastomosis to be performed. This observation is not

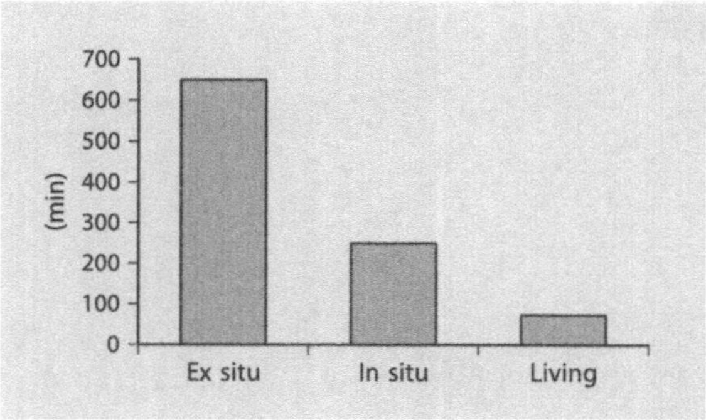

Fig. 2. Mean duration of cold ischemia time in the various harvesting procedures

unique to the venous drainage. Similar findings have been made with the arterio-portal supply to segment IV. When splitting is performed *ex situ* at the level of the falciform ligament, segment IV, which remains attached to the right graft, frequently becomes ischemic and may require primary or secondary removal [2]. In contrast, devascularization of segment IV is less frequent when the same splitting procedure is performed *in situ* [8, 9] or during living-related harvesting of the left lateral segment [13]. As experienced in our first case, a slight change in color is frequently observed just after ligation of the arterioportal pedicle to segment IV but this change improved rapidly through the development of a collateral circulation [14].

Liver function recovery was rapidly improved in patients receiving grafts harvested *in situ* as compared to those receiving *ex situ* grafts. In our experience, the liver function recovery of grafts harvested "*in situ*" was similar to grafts obtained from living-related donor.

Besides the technical considerations concerning the optimal venous drainage of the grafts, an ischemia time as short as possible is a necessary condition to achieve optimal function of the graft. This is why the *in situ* splitting and both transplantations were performed simultaneously in the same institution. As shown in Fig. 2 the mean duration of ischemia was significantly greater in cases of *ex situ* splitting as compared to *in situ* splitting. The duration of ischemia after harvesting "*in situ*" grafts was slightly higher than after resection for living-related donor.

Using a modified technique of *in situ* splitting, two adult patients can be safely transplanted with a single cadaveric graft. The basis of this modified technique is to preserve the middle hepatic vein with the left graft and the dorsal sector with the right graft and to perform splitting *in situ*, preferably without clamping of the hepatic pedicle.

The use of a graft with optimal size and quality, the availability of several teams of anesthesiologists and surgeons and the increased duration of the harvesting procedure limits the feasibility of this technique which extend the donor pool of adults.

References

1. Bismuth H, Morino M, Castaing D, Gillon MC, Descorps Declere A, Saliba F, Samuel D (1989) Emergency orthotopic liver transplantation in two patiens using one donor liver. Br J Surg 76:722–724
2. Broelsch CE, Emond JC, Whitington PF, Thistlethwaite JR, Baker AL Lichtor JL (1990) Application of reduced-size liver transplant as split graft, auxiliary orthotopic graft and living related segmental transplants. Ann Surg 212:368–377
3. Rogiers X, Malago M, Gawad K, Jauch KW, Olausson M, Knoefel WT, Glundlach M, Bassas A, Fischer L, Sterneck M, Burdelski M, Broelsch CE (1996) In situ splitting of cadaveric livers. Ann Surg 224:331–341
4. Couinaud C, Houssin D (1992) Bipartage réglé du foie en vue de transplantation. Simplification de la méthode. Chirurgie 118:217–222
5. Rela M, Vougas V, Muiesan P, Vilca-Melendez H, Smyrniotis V, Gibbs P, Karani J, Williams R, Heaton N (1998) Split liver transplantation. King's College Hospital experience. Ann Surg 227:282–288
6. Mirza DF, Achilleos O, Pirenne J, Buckels JAC, McMaster P, Mayer AD (1998) Encouraging results of split-liver transplantation. Br J Surg 85:494–497
7. Azoulay D, Astarcioglu I, Bismuth H, Castaing D, Majno P, Adam R, Johann M (1996) Split liver transplantation. The Paul Brousse policy. Ann Surg 224:737–748
8. Goss JA, Yersiz H, Shackleton CR, Seu P, Smith CV, Markowitz JS, Farmer DG, Ghobrial M (1997) In situ splitting of cadaveric liver for transplantation. Transplantation 64:871–877
9. Rogiers X, Malago M, Gawad A, Kuhlencordt R, Froshhle G, Sturm E, Sterneck M, Pothmann W (1996) One year of experience with extended application and modified techniques of split liver transplantation. Transplantation 61:1059–1061
10. Busuttil RW, Goss JA (1999) Split liver transplantation. Ann Surg 229:313–321
11. Marcos A (2000) Right lobe living donor liver transplantation: a rewiew. Liver Transplant 6:3–20
12. Colledan M, Andorno E, Valente U, Gridelli B (1999) A new splitting technique for liver grafts. Lancet 353:1763
13. Tojimbara T, Fchinoue S, Nakajima I, Koike T, Abe M, Tsugita T, Otsubo (1998) Analysis of postoperative liver function of donors in living-related liver transplantation. Transplantation 66:1035–1039
14. Sommacale D, Farges O, Ettorre GM, Lebigot P, Sauvanet A, Marty Y, Durand F, Belghiti J (2000) In situ split liver transplantation for two adult recipients. Transplantation 69:1005–1007

4 The recipient

4.1

T. Kiuchi and K. Tanaka

How much liver does the patient need?

Introduction

Considering the rapid progress in hepatology and liver surgery, it seems to be rather strange that we do not have a conclusive answer to the basic question '*How much liver does a patient need?*'. Indeed recent developments in split liver and especially living-donor liver transplantation have made significant contributions to the accumulation of knowledge for this question. It is, however, becoming clear that we have not yet obtained a final answer individualized for each patient and graft. This section tries to summarize the present information to this question, which is subject to further improvement in the near future.

How large of a liver does a healthy human have?

As the body accommodating the liver grows from infancy to adulthood, the liver rapidly increases in size and weight. After reaching a plateau in the high teens, a gradual decrease in liver weight is also reported with aging from youth to middle and old age [1]. This is attributable to the decrease of lean body mass with aging and may be modified by the nutritional status of the population defined by area and era [2]. Likewise, liver weight in males is generally greater than that in females. Furthermore, the liver to body weight ratio decreases with growth from infancy to adulthood. The liver starts with approximately 5% of body weight in infancy, and decreases and plateaus at approximately 2.5% in adults [1]. Other than age and body size, liver size can be affected by habitual intake of drugs/alcohol through enzyme induction [3,4]. Latent steatosis of the liver, which is common in the apparently healthy population, is another important factor increasing liver size unproportionally to body size.

■ How much remnant native liver does the patient need?

In the early era of liver surgery, Starzl et al. reported incomplete regeneration of remnant normal liver after extended right trisegmentectomy (85–90% resection) [5]. This case may represent a limit of resection compatible with survival. Right trisegmentectomy is generally believed to be compatible with good regeneration and survival in normal livers. In our series of lateral segment graft harvested from living donors, lateral segments, i.e., remnants after right trisegmentectomy, represent a median of 20% of the whole liver estimated by computerized tomography (CT) volumetry. However, this percentage ranges from 15 to 35% of whole liver, suggesting that a critical situation can occur in some cases after right trisegmentectomy. Within a safety limit, it is known that the regeneration rate is proportional to resected mass [6]. However, if the liver is injured with chronic hepatitis, cirrhosis, and presumably steatosis, regeneration of the remnant liver is delayed or incomplete, leading to lower survival after major hepatic resection [6, 7]. In addition to the intrinsic factors of the liver, extrahepatic complications can affect regeneration rate through extrinsic metabolic loads [8]. This information may have important implications when we consider minimum liver graft size essential for survival.

■ What impact does a small-for-size graft have in experimental animals?

In an experimental study in dogs, small-for-size liver grafts of approximately one-half size rapidly regenerated to a size equal to the original native liver with in two weeks after transplantation [9]. This implicates recipient size finally determines, at least in part, liver graft size once it is transplanted. However, another experiment, also in dogs, suggested that the minimum graft size essential for survival is at least 25–30% of the original native liver [10]. The safety limit of small-for-size grafts was more closely examined in a rodent model [11]. This experiment showed a stepwise reduction of survival as the donor-to-recipient weight ratio (D/R) decreases: 83% in D/R 1.0, 67% in D/R 0.8, 50% in D/R 0.5, and 0% in D/R 0.3. Although rodents are more sensitive to graft size mismatching than humans, the essential concept shown in experiments seems to be compatible with phenomena that we observed later in humans. However, these animal experiments almost exclusively used healthy donors and recipients and cold preservation was kept to a minimum. Therefore, it was very difficult to answer the question of how preharvesting/preservation graft injury and extrahepatic loads awaiting the graft in recipients can affect the fate of small-for-size grafts, as well as basic differences among species.

■ What have we learned from initial experiences in cadaveric or living-donor transplants?

Already in the 1980s, it was verified that small-for-size grafts transplanted into 30–60% larger recipients regenerate at a constant rate until they achieve a liver volume consistent with that expected for the given size, age and sex of the recipients [12]. In addition in the initial series of living-donor liver transplantations (LDLT), similar findings were confirmed, i.e., size of transplanted living-donor livers, 46–192% of expected liver volume, converges to expected/standard liver volume with time, regardless of small- or large-for-size grafts [13]. At this stage of optimism, the safety limit of small-for-size grafts, including variations of pretransplant metabolic debts and graft quality, was not extensively discussed.

Because a small-for-size graft has been a common concern in LDLT for larger children and adults, as well as a large-for-size graft for small babies, many LDLT programs have begun to propose their own safety criteria based on their own experiences. The proposed safety limits for small-for-size grafts were quite variable: 50% of 'standard liver volume', 40% of 'standard liver mass' or 'standard liver volume', 30% of 'standard liver volume', and 1.0% of recipient body weight [14–18]. Some reports have proposed adjustment of safety criteria to original diseases or pretransplant status, e.g., stricter criteria for cirrhotics than for non-cirrhotics, and intermediate criteria for fulminant hepatic failure [19–22], or stricter criteria for ICU-bound patients than for non-ICU-bound [18]. The smallest record of successful liver graft reported by LDLT programs ranges from 30 to 23% of 'standard liver volume' or from 0.76 to 0.59% of recipient body weight [14, 18, 19, 21–23].

■ How can we quantitate relative graft size?

There are two different ways to show graft size relative to recipient size. One is to express graft weight as percentage of expected liver size, often designated as 'standard volume', for each patient [16, 19, 21, 23, 24] and another is to express graft weight simply as percentage of recipient body weight [18, 25]. However, the methods to estimate 'standard' or 'normal' liver volume used by the former groups is not necessarily standardized. One group uses the data from autopsy cases [21] and another group uses their own data obtained from CT volumetry in the apparently healthy Japanese population [19]. Another group uses another CT volumetry in the white population, which is claimed to be different from the Japanese population [23]. Otherwise the definition of 'standard liver volume' is not clearly described [16, 24].

If the calculation or estimation of expected liver volume is based on only body surface area derived from weight and height, the obtained value would be similar to that based on only body weight. The question remains to be answered whether body size of a patient with end-stage liver disease is a sufficient information for such an estimation. Errors among different calculations would be easily surpassed by the variations of patient status and graft quality, to say nothing of variable course after transplantation. Actually the correlation of a 'standard liver volume' and simple weight ratio is acceptably good, as far as larger children and adults are concerned, and no practical problem is encountered if the same parameter is constantly applied [18,26].

■ What deleterious effects does a small-for-size graft have?

The negative impact of a small-for-size graft is not an all-or-none phenomenon. The authors reported, through a large single-center series of living-donor liver transplantations, a stepwise reduction of graft survival by the reduction of relative graft size [18]. In this series, graft survival in patients with a graft-to-recipient weight ratio (GRWR) of 1.0–3.0% was not affected by relative graft size. However, it decreased by approximately 20% when GRWR was reduced to 0.8–1.0%, and additional 20% reduction was observed when GRWR was reduced to less than 0.8%. Most graft loss in small-for-size grafts was observed by 3–6 months after transplantation. If patients were ICU-bound preoperatively, reduction of survival was more rapid.

Primary non-function was scarcely observed even in small-for-size grafts. The recovery of arterial ketone body ratio, which reflects hepatic mitochondrial energy status and serves as a good marker of primary function of liver grafts, is also excellent in small-for-size grafts. However, early posttransplant course in small-for-size grafts is eventful [18]. Transaminase release from unit graft tissue is higher in small-for-size grafts, suggesting a paradoxical hepatocyte injury despite sufficient blood flow. This is consistent with histological damage of diffuse ischemic injury and cellular ballooning [14]. Concomitantly or consequently, delayed clearance and often reincrease of cholestasis is observed in the first month after transplantation [18]. Increased incidence of surgical complications, such as intraabdominal hemorrhage or intestinal perforation, further complicates posttransplant course of small-for-size grafts, which may be a cause as well as results of initial dysfunction of small-for-size grafts.

The recent accumulation of adult cases in-living donor liver transplantation has shows similar analyses exclusively in adult patients. The negative impacts of small-for-size grafts are quite similar (Fig. 1). The peak serum bilirubin level observed several weeks after transplantation is also significantly higher in adult recipients of small-for-size grafts. The deleterious effects of small-for-size grafts are not confined to liver function tests. Not only relaparotomy from surgical complications, especially intraabdominal

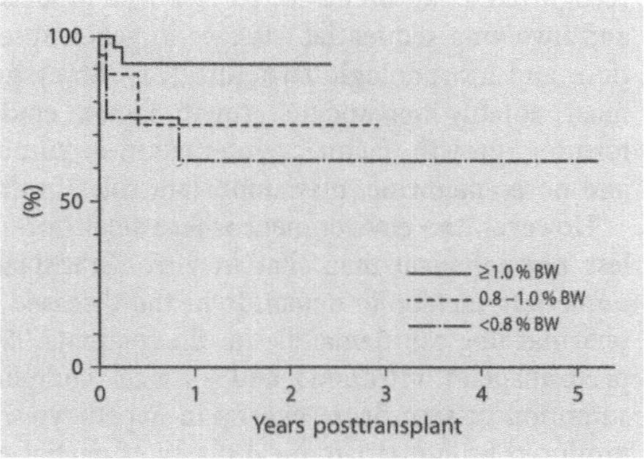

Fig. 1. Cumulative graft survival by relative graft size in 100 non-ICU-bound adult recipients of living-donor liver grafts. Graft size as percentage of recipient body weight (BW) is shown

hemorrhage, is more frequent in recipients of small-for-size grafts, but also more bacteremia is observed especially in adult patients with small-for-size grafts. This may support the concept that transplanted liver play an important role in infection immunity in the recipients. Interestingly, serum creatinine level, which is often transiently elevated, especially in the adult population after liver transplantation due to water imbalance and many renotoxic drugs, is significantly higher in recipients of small-for-size grafts, suggesting some hepatorenal effect of graft size.

Negative impacts of small-for-size grafts are also strongly modified by pretransplant status or original diseases. Impact is rather small in patients who had almost full activity before transplantation. Fulltime bed-bound patients, however, suffer much larger negative impacts of small-for-size grafts. Even in ICU-bound patients, those with chronic illness, i.e., status 2a in UNOS criteria, suffer much larger impacts of small-for-size grafts than those with acute illness as status 1, suggesting that metabolic debts in status 2a patients are much larger than those in status 1 patients as far as graft size is concerned. In addition, reduction of graft survival by reduction of graft size is larger in cirrhotics than in non-cirrhotics. Actually our personal record of successful smallest-for-size graft is only 0.47% of body weight (23% of 'standard liver volume'), which was implanted into a 30-year-old patient with familial amyloidotic polyneuropathy. As well as patient factors, graft factors, e.g., steatosis, preservation/reperfusion injury, or graft injury after transplantation, can reduce functional volume of grafts and aggravate the negative impact of small-for-size grafts.

■ Why do small-for-size liver grafts fail? A hypothesis

Liver regeneration after the loss of hepatic tissue is a fundamental response of the liver to injury. A similar response is also expected in small-for-size grafts placed into a new environment. This phenomenon is now recognized as an orchestrated response induced by specific external stimuli and involving sequential changes in gene expression, growth factor production, and morphologic structure [27]. Many growth factors and cytokines, most notably hepatocyte growth factor, epidermal growth factor, transforming growth factor-*α*, interleukin-6, tumor necrosis factor-*α*, insulin and norepinephrine, play important roles in this process.

However, the environment where small-for-size grafts are placed is much less physiological than that in vitro. Transplanted liver is obliged to face numerous metabolic demands in the diseased host as well as surgical and pharmacological demands in the patients. Metabolic load produced by peritransplant infectious and surgical complications may lead to a consumption of significant energy in hepatocytes. Also non-functioning tissue produced by non-anatomical plasty of partial grafts may act as a metabolic load on functioning hepatocytes. On the other hand, variations in functional reserve of partial liver grafts, partly attributable to preharvesting occult abnormalities, preservation/reperfusion injuries, and immunological injuries after transplantation, are much larger than expected even in living-donor grafts.

As a consequence of the balance among these complicated factors, energy metabolism in hepatic mitochondria is conjectured to decline to a minus, leading to the failure in signal transduction in hepatocytes and in sequential orchestration. We have experienced that small-for-size grafts that eventually failed did not necessarily fail to regenerate as far as macroscopic size is concerned. Abnormal morphology observed in small-for-size grafts may represent an abnormal growth or regeneration of the grafts. Loss of sequential coordination among proliferations in hepatocytes, biliary ductular cells, Kupffer and Ito cells, and sinusoidal endothelial cells, might also play a role [27].

■ How can we predict the size of the partial liver graft?

Apart from the impact of small-for-size grafts, a more practical problem is that we have not yet obtained a good way to predict precisely the size of the partial liver graft from cadaveric donors. In the living-donor program, the elective situation permits the estimation of anatomical graft size by CT volumetry. The predictability of CT volumetry is excellent and the error is usually within 5%. However, such a method is not applicable for cadaveric donors, with rare exceptions. Data from the living-donor program shows that the variation of graft size even in the same anatomical lobes from donors with the same body weight is much larger than expected (Fig. 2b). The principle of 1.5% or 1.0% of body weight for the right or left lobe of the liver is hardly true in harvested graft weight. Furthermore, the use of body surface area, instead of body weight, scarcely amends the situation (Fig. 2a).

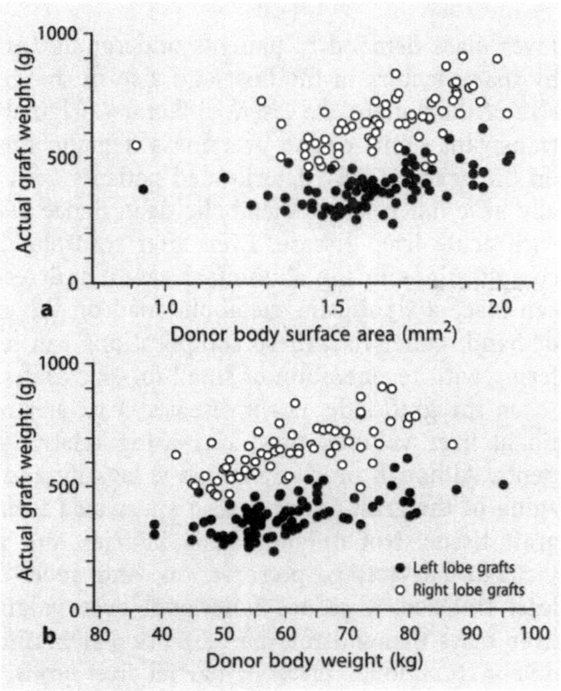

Fig. 2. Relationship between donor body surface area (**a**) or donor body weight (**b**) and actual liver graft weight harvested from living donors

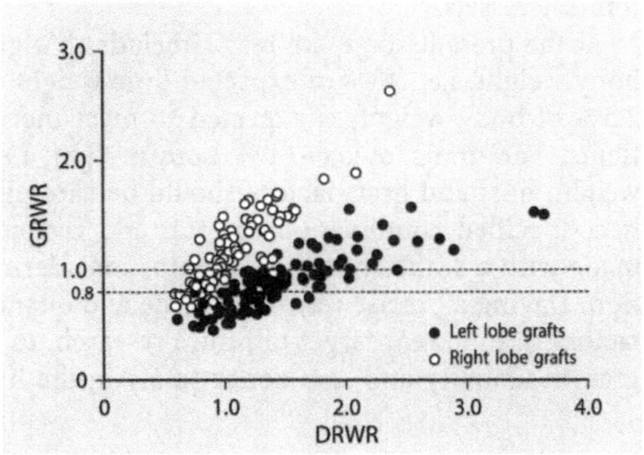

Fig. 3. Relationship between donor-to-recipient weight ratio (DRWR) and resultant graft-to-recipient weight ratio (GRWR, shown in %) in living-donor liver transplantation using the left lobe (with middle hepatic vein, without caudate lobes) and right lobe (without middle hepatic vein) grafts

A practical method would be to know the possible minimum GRWR in the given donor-to-recipient weight ratio (Fig. 3). If a donor has a weight similar to that of the recipient, the right lobe graft obtained from the donor serves GRWR of 1.0% in most cases. For a left lobe graft to be 1.0% of recipient body weight with certainty, donor weight should be more than twice the recipient's weight.

Conclusions – what can we say at the present stage?

Liver mass demand in patients undergoing transplantation can be affected by many factors in the host and also in the graft. Although age and body size of the patient are essential factors, original diseases and especially pre-transplant status define liver mass demand through metabolic load placed on the graft. Highly deteriorated patients with chronic liver disease generally have much larger metabolic debt, hence liver mass demand, than those with acute liver disease. Even after transplantation, surgical or infectious complications in the abdominal cavity and resultant prolonged cholestasis can place a significant metabolic load on the graft and increase liver mass demand. Otherwise, these complications can lead to a vicious circle interfering with regeneration of small-for-size grafts.

On the graft side, latent diseases, e.g., steatosis or fibrosis, reduce functional liver volume, thus, increasing relative liver mass demand for patients. Although precise analysis is lacking and the variation may be large, aging of the graft donor is also speculated to impose similar effects on the graft tissue. Not only intrinsic injuries, but also extrinsic graft injuries through harvesting, preservation, and reperfusion procedures would, at least transiently, reduce functional liver volume, thus, increasing relative liver mass demand for the patients. Furthermore, an important factor reducing functional mass in partial liver graft is the possible presence of non-functioning tissue adjacent to the transection plane, which is potentially derived from ischemia or congestion through the deprivation of anatomical vessels.

At the present stage, we may conclude that graft size of more than 1% of body weight, i.e., 40% of expected liver weight if the liver is assumed to be 2.5% of body weight, is expected to meet metabolic demands in most patients. For grafts of 0.6–1.0% body weight, i.e. 25–40% of expected liver weight, host and graft factors should be carefully evaluated to calculate risk in a specified combination of graft and recipient. The decision should be made with a sufficient safety margin, considering possible errors in estimation. Having a precise way to estimate and quantitate graft and recipient risk factors is an urgent target of future research, to maximize patient safety and graft availability and also donor safety in the living-donor program.

References

1. Aimi S, Yasoshima S, Sugai M, Sato B, Sakai T, Nakajima Y (1952) Studies on the weight and size of internal organs of normal Japanese. Acta Pathol Jap 2:173–200
2. Van Thiel DH, Gavaler JS, Kam I et al (1987) Rapid growth of an intact human liver transplanted into a recipient larger than the donor. Gastroenterology 93:1414–1419

3. Reichel C, Block W, Skodra T et al (1997) Relationship between cytochrome P-450 induction by rifampicin, hepatic volume and portal flow in man. Eur J Gastroenterol Hepatol 9:975–979
4. Blomquist L, Wang Y, Kimiaei S, Jacobsson H (1994) Change in size, shape and radiocolloid uptake of the alcoholic liver during alcohol withdrawal, as demonstrated by single photon emission computed tomography. J Hepatol 21:417–423
5. Starzl TE, Putnam CW, Groth CG, Corman JL, Taubman J (1975) Alopecia, ascites, and incomplete regeneration after 85–90 per cent liver resection. Am J Surg 129:587–590
6. Yamanaka N, Okamoto E, Kawamura E et al (1993) Dynamics of normal and injured human liver regeneration after hepatectomy as assessed on the basis of computed tomography and liver function. Hepatology 18:79–85
7. Chen MF, Hwang TL, Hung CF (1991) Human liver regeneration after major hepatectomy: a study of liver volume by computed tomography. Ann Surg 213:227–229
8. Szawlowski AW, Faurous P, Saint-Aubert B et al (1986) Single photon emission computerized tomography (SPECT) for monitoring regeneration of the human liver after partial hepatectomy for secondary tumours. Eur J Surg Oncol 12: 389–392
9. Kam I, lynch S, Svanas G et al (1987) Evidence that host size determines liver size: studies in dogs receiving orthotopic liver transplants. Hepatology 7:362–366
10. Shirakata Y, Terajima H, Mashima S, et al (1995) The minimum graft size for successful orthotopic partial liver transplantation in the canine model. Transplant Proc 27:545–546
11. Xu HS, Pruett TL, Jones RS (1994) Study of donor-recipient liver size match for transplantation. Ann Surg 219:46–50
12. Van Thiel DH, Gavaler JS, Kam I et al (1987) Rapid growth of an intact human liver transplanted into a recipient larger than the donor. Gastroenterology 93:1414–1419
13. Kawasaki S, Makuuchi M, Ishizone S, Matsunami H, Terada M, Kawarazaki H (1992) Liver regeneration in recipients and donors after transplantation. Lancet 339:580–581
14. Emond JC, Renz JF, Ferrell LD et al (1996) Functional analysis of grafts from living donors: implications for the treatment of older recipients. Ann Surg 244:544–552
15. Furukawa H, Kishida A, Omura T et al (1999) Indication and strategy for adult living related liver transplantation. Transplant Proc 31:1952
16. Park KM, Lee SG, Lee YJ et al (1999) Adult-to-adult living donor liver transplantation at Asan Medical Center, Seoul, Korea. Transplant Proc 31:456–458
17. Harihara Y, Makuuchi M, Kawasaki H et al (1999) Initial experience with 40 cases of living-related donor liver transplantation at the University of Tokyo. Transplant Proc 31:2893–2894
18. Kiuchi T, Kasahara M, Uryuhara K et al (1999) Impact of graft size mismatching on graft prognosis in liver transplantation from living donors. Transplantation 67:321–327
19. Kawasaki S, Makuuchi M, Matsunami H et al (1998) Living related liver transplantation in adults. Ann Surg 227:269–274
20. Miwa S, Hashikura Y, Mita A et al (1999) Living-related liver transplantation for patients with fulminant and subfulminant hepatic failure. Hepatology 30:1521–1526

21. Lo CM, Fan ST, Chan JK et al (1996) Minimum graft volume for successful adult-to-adult living donor liver transplantation for fulminant hepatic failure. Transplantation 62:696–698
22. Lo CM, Fan ST, Liu CL et al (1999) Minimum graft size for successful living donor liver transplantation. Transplantation 68:1112–1116
23. Heinemann A, Wischhusen F, Puschel K, Rogiers X (1999) Standard liver volume in the Caucasian population. Liver Transpl Surg 5:366–368
24. Wachs ME, Bak TE, Karrer FM et al (1998) Adult living donor liver transplantation using a right hepatic lobe. Transplantation 66:1313–1316
25. Marcos A, Fisher RA, Ham JM et al (1999) Right lobe living donor liver transplantation. Transplantation 68:798–803
26. Marcos A (2000) Right lobe living donor liver transplantation: a review. Liver Transplant 6:3–20
27. Michalopoulos GK, DeFrances MC (1997) Liver regeneration. Science 276:60–66

4.2

M. GUNDLACH, S. TOPP, D. C. BROERING, and X. ROGIERS

Transplantation of the right liver graft – technical aspects

■ Introduction

The transplantation of segmental grafts from cadaveric and living donors usually requires a vena cava-preserving recipient hepatectomy to allow the implantation of the donor liver. Only split grafts, preserving the donor vena cava are as well transplantable in traditional fashion with end-to-end anastomosis of the infra- and suprahepatic caval vein.

Calne in 1968 and Tzakis in 1989 described the piggyback technique with preservation of the recipient vena cava and direct anastomosis of the donor's vena cava with the recipient's hepatic veins [1, 2]. The technique of filleting the diseased liver from the recipients inferior vena cava (IVC), followed by partial clamping of the IVC at the level of the hepatic veins allows caval flow during the anhepatic phase. By using this technique venovenous bypass can be avoided [2, 3].

In split liver transplantation for one adult and one child, the right graft usually retained the vena cava, the common bile duct, the portal trunk and the right hepatic artery. The common hepatic artery with the coeliac trunk stayed with the left graft. Right lobe implantation is therefore similar to a whole liver transplantation. The main trunk of the portal vein, right hepatic artery and common bile duct are available for anastomosis. A duct to duct biliary anastomosis is usually possible, provided that there is an intact blood supply from the right hepatic artery.

■ Engraftment of right liver graft after "piggyback" hepatectomy

The increasing use of partial liver grafts modified the techniques of hepato-venous reconstruction and the number of anastomosis has been reduced since the piggyback technique has become a standard procedure in clinical liver transplantation. Before hepatectomy of the diseased liver, the vena cava is partially clamped below or at the level of the hepatic veins.

The engraftment of the extended right donor liver should begin with reconstruction of the hepato-venous outflow. Several different techniques in split liver transplantation has been described:

- Direct anastomosis of the donor's vena cava with the recipient's main hepatic veins (classical "piggyback"-technique) [1, 2]
- End-to-side cavocavostomy [4]
- Side-to-side caval anastomosis [5].

In case of end-to-side or side-to-side cavocavosomy, all hepatic veins of the recipient are sutured and cavo-caval anastomosis is performed as described below.

At the University Hospital Eppendorf in Hamburg a combined technique is used for hepato-venous outflow reconstruction. During piggyback hepatectomy the recipient‘s right hepatic vein is dissected and sutured. The vena cava is partially clamped at the level of the recipient‘s hepatic veins. Before engraftment of the donor liver, the orifice of the middle and left hepatic veins are opened and extended along the frontwall of the recipient‘s vena cava to produce a large triangle.

The donor IVC is distally closed, followed by longitudinal incision of the backwall. The vena cava is then anastomosed side-to-side in a wide venacavoplasty with a running 4/0 prolene suture. The anastomosis is left open to allow the albumin flush via the portal vein at completion of venacavoplasty.

In split liver transplantation for two adult recipients, the donor liver has to be split through the midplane to provide enough liver mass for both recipients. Usually the middle hepatic vein is retained with the left and the vena cava with the right split graft. The indispensable division of the caudate lobe veins lead to uncertain viability of liver segment I and resection might be necessary. To maintain all retrohepatic veins for optimal venous drainage of both grafts, we recently developed the split cava technique [6]. This split technique results in two grafts, each with a large venous patch including both the main hepatic vein and additional smaller retrohepatic veins draining it. Implantation of the grafts is performed using a standard technique with a side-to-side cavocavostomy [7].

The adequate reconstruction of afferent vessels is a precondition for successful liver transplantation. Poor blood inflow and technical problems often lead to early postoperative organ failure and graft loss. The determination of the preoperative vascular status of both the recipient and the donor organ is necessary for optimal transplant re-vascularization due to the multitude of arterial variants and pathological changes in the afferent liver vasculature, like thrombosis or stenosis.

The standard portal vein reconstruction is an end-to-end anastomosis between the donor and recipient portal vein, with a continuous 5/0 or 6/0 prolene suture leaving a growth factor of about one-third of the diameter of the vessel to avoid stenosis. Before closure of the cavocaval and the portal anastomosis, the liver is flushed usually with 20% albumin via the portal vein.

A normal portal bifurcation is present in 80% of grafts and other variations tend to involve the right branch of the portal vein in about 20–30%. Absence of the right branch is the most common anomaly with a trifurcation of the main trunk. In this situation the main portal vein trunk should be kept in continuity with the right lobe graft. Pathological modifications, like portal vein thrombosis or cavernous transformation cause a portal anastomosis at the confluence of the recipient portal vein with or without interposition of vein grafts. Portal venous reconstruction of the right lobe graft should be performed using a donor iliac vein.

The arterial graft supply as well as anatomical circumstances of the recipient determines the method of arterial reconstruction. A number of arterial variations and proposed methods of reconstruction have been described [8]. Essentially for engraftment is the determination whether there is a sole arterial supply for the right graft or if there is an additional branch from the superior mesenteric artery. The ideal arrangement is a simple division of the common hepatic artery which is present in 50% of livers. The right hepatic artery in these organs is invariably larger than the left branch and should therefore be divided. In approximately 10% the right hepatic artery arises from the superior mesenteric artery as sole supply for the right graft [9]. Arterial duplications occur more commonly on the left. In 25% of potential grafts, the left hepatic artery divides into two branches and in 1% of organs there is a trifurcation. In general the common hepatic artery should be kept in continuity on the side with the arterial duplication. In liver donations with long arteries, the vessels are usually shortened to the common hepatic artery for reconstruction.

The arterial anastomosis between the right hepatic artery, with or without the donor truncus, and the hepatic arteria in the area of the gastroduodenal artery passage is usually performed as arterial reconstruction. The object of this anastomosis is the expansion of the arterial circle and to supply the donor artery from the hepatic and superior mesenteric artery of the recipient.

If possible, the hepatic artery is anastomosed using a branch patch technique [10, 11]. The anastomosis is performed with either an interrupted or a continuous 6/0 or 7/0 prolene suture. If the artery is small a modified microvascular technique of interrupted sutures is used.

Once hemostasis is established the biliary anastomosis may be reconstructed. A direct duct-to-duct anastomosis using 6/0 PDS suture is usually performed with or without insertion of a T-drain. It is important to trim the ends of both the ducts particularly on the donor side to ensure a good blood supply. A Roux-en-Y hepaticojejunostomy is performed in all cases of sclerosing cholangitis and in concern over the quality and caliber of the bile ducts. Usually a length of 40 cm is used.

Before abdominal closure, complete hemostasis should be secured. The liver should be lifted forward and the retrohepatic areas and all anastomoses carefully examined. Especially the transection margin should be carefully inspected to detect bleeding points and visible bile leaks.

Conclusion

"Piggyback" transplantation with side-to-side cavocavostomy is an ideal technique for extended right split liver graft implantation. Experience with adult piggyback implantation using a side-to-side cavocavostomy resulted in a modification of the implantation of the extended right split lobe.

Using the classical technique of piggyback liver implantation, with anastomosis between suprahepatic inferior vena cava cuff and hepatic vein cuff of the recipient, may be difficult. Some torsion or stenosis of this anastomosis, caused by compression of hepatic veins may occur when the right hepatic lobe falls down into its fossa.

The longitudinal cavotomy along the backwall of the donors vena cava together with an opening of the hepatic vein orifices easily allows a latero-lateral anastomosis of the recipient's and donor's vena cava. Our technique provides optimal venous drainage of the right and middle hepatic vein and all retrohepatic veins, avoiding congestion and thus extensive bleeding at the right hepatic lobe transection margin [12].

To date, specific complications of a cava preserving transplantation technique are poorly reported in the literature. Large series of piggyback transplantation identified two major complications: hemorrhage and occlusion of the caval venous return or Budd-Chiary syndrome [4]. The incidence of these complications correlates with the surgical technique of venuous outflow reconstruction. The incidence of venous outflow occlusion is significantly increased after classic "piggyback" implantation [4]. The technique related congestion may also lead to increased postoperative ascites production, due to portal hypertension [13].

In summary, the engrafment of the extended right split graft does not differ considerably from whole organ liver transplantation. In our experience the implantation of the right graft using a wide side-to-side cavocavostomy is technically feasible, without an increased postoperative complication rate.

References

1. Calne RY, Williams R (1968) Liver transplantation in man: observations on technique and organization in 5 cases. BMJ 4:535
2. Tzakis A, Todo S, Starzl TE (1989) Orthotopic liver transplantation with preservation of the inferior vena cava. Ann Surg 210:649
3. Bismuth H, Castaing D, Sherlog DJ (1990) Liver transplantation by 'face-a-face' venacavaplasty. Surgery 111:151–155
4. Navarro F, Le Moine MC, Fabre JM, Belghiti DC, et al. (1999) Specific vascular complications of orthotopic liver transplantation with preservation of the retrohepatic vena cava: review of 1361 cases. Transplantation 68:646–650

5. Belghiti J, Panis Y, Sauvanet A, Gayet B, Fekete F (1992) A new technique of side to side caval anastomosis during orthotopic hepatic transplantation without inferior vena caval clamping. Surg Gynocol Obst 175:270
6. M Gundlach, DC Broering, S Topp, M Sterneck, X Rogiers (2000) Split-cava technique: liver splitting for two adult recipients. Liver Transplantation 6(6): 703–706
7. Lerut J, de Ville de Goyet, Donataccio M, Reding R, Otte JB (1994) Piggyback transplantation with side-to-side cavocavostomy is an ideal technique for right split liver allograft implantation. J Am Coll Surg 179:573–576
8. Shaw BW, Wood RP, Stratta RJ, et al. (1990) Management of arterial anomalies encountered in split-liver transplantation. Transplant Proc 22:420–422
9. Daseler EH, Anson BJ, Hambley WC, Reimann AF (1947) The cystic artery and the constituents of the hepatic pedicle. Surgery 85:47–63
10. Quinones-Baldrich WJ, Memsic L, Ramming K, Hiatt J, Busuttil RW (1986) Branch patch for arterialisation of hepatic grafts. Surgery 162:489–491
11. Kalayoglu M, Belzer O (1987) A new technique for arterialisation of the hepatic graft. Surg Gynocol Obst 164:564–567
12. Houssin D, Boillot O, Soubrane O, et al. (1993) Controlled liver splitting for transplantation in two recipients: technique, results and perspectives. Br J Surg 80:75–80
13. Cirera I, Navasa M, Rimola A, et al. (2000) Ascites after liver transplantation. Liver Transplant 6(2):157–162

4.3 B. Gridelli

B. Gridelli

Technique of implantation of the left graft

■ Introduction

The split liver technique was originally devised to transplant children without discarding the excess liver parenchyma, which could be used to transplant an adult patient [1]. From this operation, which can be performed *ex situ* or *in situ* [2], derives a left graft constituted by segments II and III, or left lateral segment (LLS), and a right graft constituted by segments I and IV to VIII of Couinaud. Despite initial unsatisfactory results, the effort to render split liver transplantation an effective way to meet the needs of children for liver grafts without interfering with the adult waiting list continued, particularly, in Europe. The results of this effort are such that split liver transplantation has become a common practice in several centers around the world. In particular, the techniques of implantation of the LLS have reached a high degree of maturity which has its roots in nearly twenty years of experience with reduced-size liver transplantation.

New techniques of liver splitting with the aim of transplanting two adult patients with one liver, have been devised [3–5]. Depending on the different techniques, the division of the liver, performed *in situ* or *ex situ*, generates two different sets of grafts. The left one can be constituted by segments I to IV along with the vena cava, or II to IV without the vena cava, and the right by segments V to VIII, or I plus V to VIII along with the vena cava.

■ Techniques of implantation of the LLS

The vascular components of the LLS vary according to the anatomy and the division techniques used. To describe the techniques of implantation, the order of the vascular anastomosis performed during the operation will be followed.

Hepatic vein anastomosis

Segments II and III usually drain into the vena cava through a single left hepatic vein that can be directly anastomosed to the recipient vena cava. The anastomosis can be performed between a cuff of the left and middle hepatic vein or the right hepatic vein of the recipient and the left hepatic vein of the graft [6, 7]. These types of anastomosis are at risk of stricture and kinking, which can result in an outflow obstruction. In its most severe and acute form, an outflow obstruction can result in graft failure requiring emergency retransplantation to rescue the patient. Milder, more chronic forms of outflow obstruction usually become evident in the days and weeks after transplantation with production of large quantities of ascites and/or pleural effusion. Usually, in these situations, the outflow obstruction can be relieved by percutaneous balloon dilatation of the stenotic anastomosis.

To reduce the risk of outflow obstruction, Emond devised a triangulation technique of suprahepatic vein reconstruction in reduced-size liver transplantation [8], which is probably the safest and most commonly used technique in implantation of LLS (Figs. 1, 2).

In children with liver tumors, it is oncologically sound to remove the vena cava along with the native liver. In two cases, we replaced the infrahepatic vena cava, sewing to the graft left hepatic vein a donor iliac vein on the back table.

Portal vein anastomosis

The trunk of the portal vein can be retained either with the left or right hepatic graft. We usually leave the portal trunk with the right graft. The portal vein reconstruction in the recipient can be performed in four differ-

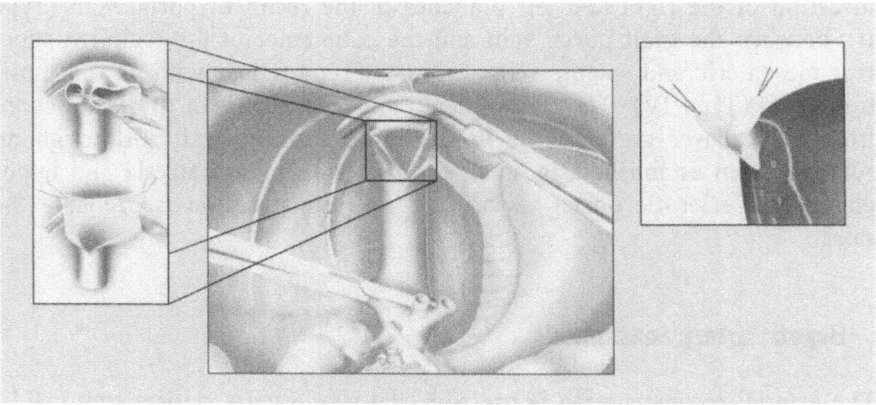

Fig. 1. On the front wall of the recipient vena cava a wide triangular opening is prepared joining together the three hepatic veins (modified from Emon, 1993)

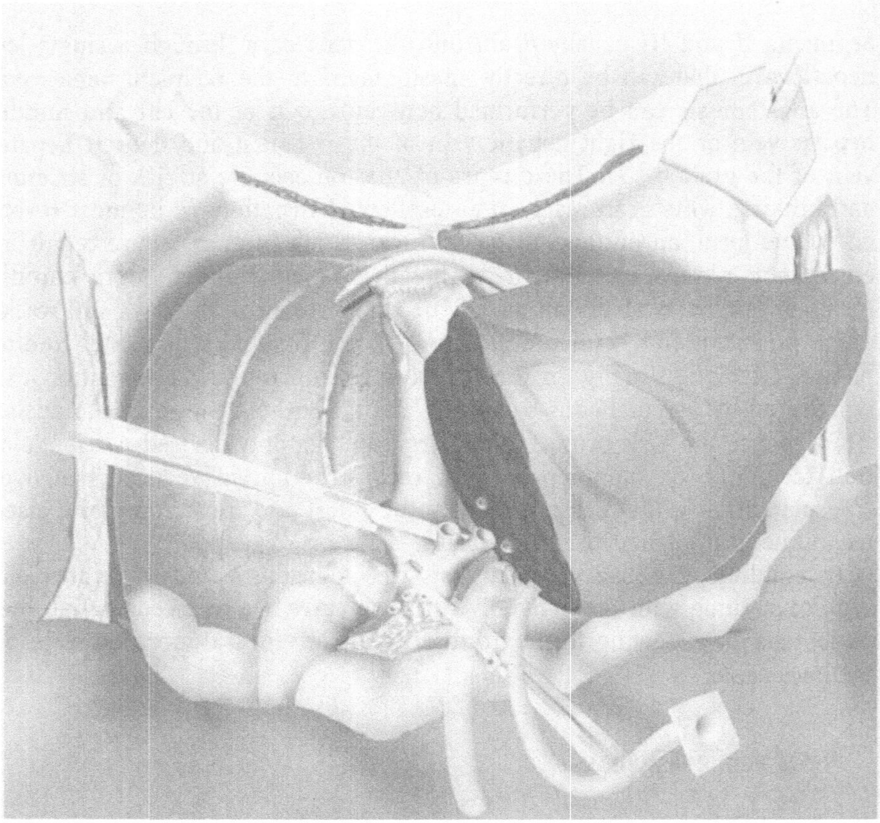

Fig. 2. The left hepatic vein of the graft is sutured, with the triangulation technique, to the recipient vena cava. During the anastomosis, the liver is flushed from the preservation solution.

ent ways [9]: end-to-end (Type I), between the graft portal vein and the bifurcation of the right and left branches of the recipient portal vein (Type II), between the graft portal vein and the confluence of the recipient superior mesenteric and splenic veins, without (Type III) or with an interposition graft (Type IV). The iliac, splenic and superior vein grafts procured from the cadaver graft can be used as interposition grafts. Although no rule has been established, in small children with biliary atresia and hypoplastic and sclerotic portal veins, Type IV reconstruction is probably the safest.

Hepatic artery anastomosis

The arterial reconstruction is probably the single most critical step in LLS implantation. Arterial thrombosis, the most feared technical complication, has been reported after implantation of the left graft deriving from splitting the liver, with rates from 0 up to 25% in the earliest series. When splitting the liver, the celiac trunk can either be retained with the right or left graft. Upon implantation, the arterial reconstruction can be obtained by anastomosing the graft arterial supply directly to the recipient hepatic artery, if of appropriate size, or to the aorta with or without an interposition graft. Inomoto [10] has extensively described the microsurgical techniques used to reconstruct the hepatic artery in living-related liver transplantation; similar techniques should be used when the LLS from split liver is procured along with the left hepatic artery.

Biliary tract anastomosis

The reconstruction of the LLS biliary tract is obtained via a Roux en-Y hepaticojejunostomy; in over 20% of the cases there are two separate bile ducts for segments II and III which have to be anastomosed individually. Complications in the bile duct reconstruction are frequent and can be represented by stricture or leak; these complications have been reported with incidences as high as 40% in the early series. Most centers performing split liver and living-related liver transplantation report incidences of biliary complications between 10 and 20%, although series with much lower biliary complications have been published by Rogiers and Busuttil [11, 12]. One way to reduce biliary complications is to use a proper technique of splitting: it is important to sharply cut the left hilar plate and to tie the small bile ducts encountered during the parenchymal transection to avoid biliary leaks from the cut surface.

■ Implantation of the full left graft

In 1989 Bismuth had already reported the *ex situ* splitting of one liver for transplantation of two adult recipients [13]. The idea of using one liver for two adults was resurrected in 1999 [3], and various techniques of *ex situ* and *in situ* splitting have been described. Depending on the technique used the left graft is constituted of segments II to IV without the vena cava or segments I to IV with the vena cava. We have chosen to divide the liver *in situ* leaving the vena cava and segment I, which represent 8–10% of the mass of the left hemiliver, with the left graft which can then be transplanted exactly like a whole liver. Other groups implant the left graft, constituted by segments II to IV, with the piggyback technique. The left biliary duct must be anastomosed to a Roux en-Y jejunal loop and particular care must be paid to identify the small bile duct on the wide cut surface to reduce the incidence of leaks both during the donor operation and after implantation.

■ The Bergamo experience

The Liver Transplant Center of the Ospedali Riuniti of Bergamo, which started its activity in October 1997, implemented an active program of *in situ* split liver transplantation for children in collaboration with other Italian transplant centers transplanting adult patients only. No donor upper age limit was established for acceptance in the split liver program and livers from donors as old as 65 years have been successfully divided and transplanted. After 2.5 years of activity, 94 pediatric liver transplants have been performed in Bergamo, 85 were primary transplants and 9 retransplants (10.5%), two of which in patients who had been transplanted elsewhere and had developed chronic rejection. Sixty-two were split liver transplants (65.9%), 24 (25.5%) were whole and 8 (8.5%) reduced-size liver transplants. Over 60% of the patients were below two years of age. The median time on the waiting list was 22 days and there was no mortality before transplantation. The actuarial survival of all the patients and grafts at one year is 89% and 81%, respectively. The one-year patient and graft survival in the split liver group is 90% and 88%, respectively. At the beginning of our experience we had one acute outflow obstruction in a patient receiving a LLS from split liver. The child was retransplanted within 24 hours with an incompatible graft from a split liver and is alive and well at two years posttransplantation. No patient receiving LLS from split livers experienced arterial thrombosis, while in 4 patients (8.0%) an ultrasound diagnosis of portal vein thrombosis was made. In two patients the revision of the anastomosis was performed, one patient (a 40-day-old child weighing 3 kg with fulminant liver failure who was transplanted with a LLS from a 75 kg donor) died 30 days posttransplant because of sepsis, the other is alive and well over one year after the transplant. The two remaining children in whom portal vein thrombosis did not have any clinical manifestation were only observed and are alive and well 8 and 6 months posttransplantation with no sign of portal hypertension nor of hypersplenism.

Complications at the biliary reconstruction developed in 8 patients (12.9%). Six patients had anastomotic strictures that in 4 cases were successfully treated with percutaneous balloon dilatation and in 2 with reoperation. In two patients anastomotic leaks were treated with reoperation; bile leaks from the cut surface were treated with percutaneous drainage in 4 patients. No patient or graft was lost because of biliary complications.

Three patients, aged 13, 10 and 21 years with body weights of 48, 38 and 55 kg, were transplanted with a full left graft (segments I to IV along with the vena cava). They are alive and well 14, 10 and 8 months after transplantation, respectively. The third patient was retransplanted with a whole liver 8 days after the first transplant because of arterial thrombosis.

Conclusion

The procurement and implantation of LLS from split livers is a safe and effective way of transplanting children without penalizing adult patients. The techniques of vascular reconstruction have reached a high degree of standardization, and patient and graft loss due to vascular complications can be virtually eliminated; although biliary complications are still a problem in most centers, most of the times they can easily be dealt with by interventional radiology or reoperation. The newer techniques of liver splitting which aim at using one liver for two adults will probably reach the same degree of efficacy in the next few years. We believe the full left graft should be constituted by segments I to IV along with the vena cava, providing the maximum possible liver mass.

Split liver transplantation, and in particular the *in situ* technique, has completely changed the outlook for children needing liver replacement and their families. It is possible that the evolution of liver splitting for two adults will provide a significant reduction of the shortage of grafts for adult patients.

References

1. Pichlmayr R, Ringe B, Gubernatis G, et al. (1998) Transplantation einer Spenderleber auf zwei Empfänger (Splitting-Transplantation) – Eine neue Methode in der Weiterentwicklung der Lebersegmenttransplantation. Langenbecks Arch Chir 373: 127
2. Rogiers X, Malago M, Habib N, et al. (1995) In situ splitting of the liver in the heart-beating cadaveric organ donor for transplantation in two recipients. Transplantation 59:1081–1083
3. Colledan M, Andorno E, Valente U, et al. (1999) A new splitting technique for liver grafts. Lancet 353:1763
4. Azoulay D, Castaing D, Adam R, et al. (2000) Transplantation of three adult patients with one cadaveric graft: wait or innovate. Liver Transplantation 6:239–240
5. Sommacle D, Farges O, Ettorre GM, et al. (2000) In situ split liver transplantation for two adult recipients. Transplantation 69:1005–1007
6. Emond JC, Whitington PF, Thistlethwaite JR, et al. (1989) Transplantation of two patients with one liver. Ann Surg 212:14–22
7. Otte JB, de Ville de Goyet J, Alberti D, et al. (1990) The concept and technique of the split liver in clinical transplantation. Surgery 6:605–612
8. Emond JC, Heffron TG, Whitington PF, et al. (1993) Reconstruction of the hepatic vein in reduced size hepatic transplantation. Surg Gynecol Obstet 176: 11–17
9. Saad S, Tanaka K, Inomata Y, et al. (1998) Portal vein reconstruction in pediatric liver transplantation from living donors. Ann Surg 2:275–281

10. Inomoto T, Nishizawa F, Sasaki H, et al. (1996) Experiences of 120 microsurgical reconstructions of hepatic artery in living related liver transplantation. Surgery 119:20–26
11. Rogiers X, Malagò M, Gawad K, et al. (1996) In situ splitting of cadaveric livers. The ultimate expansion of a limited donor pool. Ann Surg 224:331–341
12. Busuttil RW, Goss JA (1999) Split liver transplantation. Ann Surg 229:313–321
13. Bismuth H, Morino M, Castaing D, et al. (1989) Emergency orthotopic liver transplantation in two patients using one liver. Br J Surg 76:722–724

5 Results and outlook

5.1

S. Topp, D.C. Broering, and X. Rogiers

Results of *ex situ* split liver transplantation

Since the introduction of SLT in 1988, more than 400 documented *ex situ* SLT have been performed worldwide. Table 1 provides an overview of the results through 2000 [1–14].

The initial results of SLT were disappointing in comparison to those obtained from whole and reduced grafts. The reported graft and patient survival were 50% and 43%, respectively [3, 4]. Because of this, the procedure was initially not considered suitable for elective patients and did not generate enthusiastic support at its inception. The idea of transplanting two different recipients with two segmental grafts from one donor liver appeared technically challenging (Fig. 1) and was associated with prolonged cold ischemia times (Fig. 2).

Table 1. Published experience with *ex situ* split liver grafts for adults and children (*BC* biliary complications, *VC* vascular complications)

Author	Year	Number of *ex situ* SLT	Survival rate (%)		BC (%)	VC (%)
			patient	graft		
Emond [2]	1990	18	67	50	27	6
Broelsch [3]	1990	30	50	43	27	
Otte [4]	1990	4	50	50		
Sloof [5]	1995	15	73	67		
Otte [6]	1995	29	71	67	17.2	10.3
De Ville [7]	1995	98	68	62	23	10.2
Rogiers [8]	1996	19	63	58	16	
Kalayoglu [9]	1996	12	91	75	25	
Mirza [10]	1998	24	78	68	12.5	8.3
Rela [1]	1998	41	90	88	14.6	4.9
Sindhy [11]	1999	89	82	60.3		
Chardot [12]	1999	16	66.7	62.5	25	43.7
Rogiers [13]	1999	29	75.5	72.3	10.3	6.9
Reyes [14]	2000	24	74	60	8	16

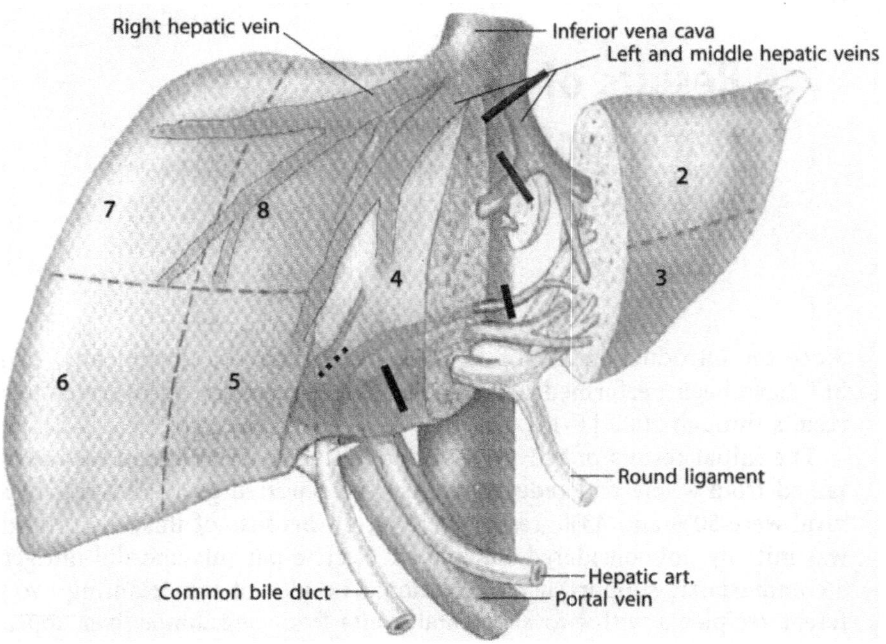

Fig. 1. Splitting the liver just as a formal left lateral segmentectomy (II/III) provides an extended right lobe and a left lateral segment graft for transplantation of one adult and one child. — Cutting lines; - - - dependent on the arterial anatomy the hepatic artery could be cut alternatively on the right side, retaining the truncus with the left lateral graft

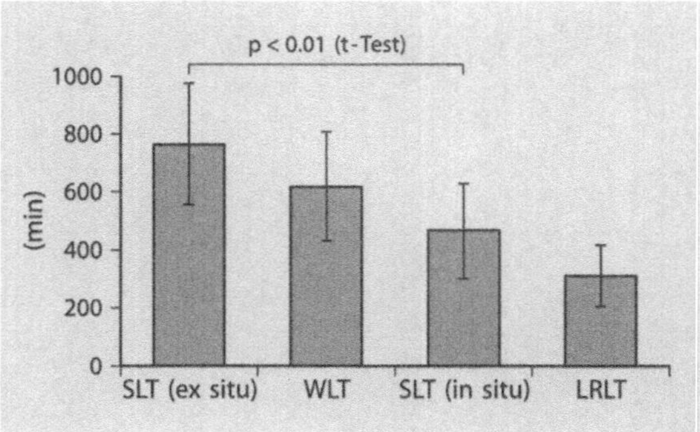

Fig. 2. Mean cold ischemia times of liver transplantation in Hamburg (1993–1999). *WLT* whole liver transplantation (n=582), *SLT* split liver transplantation (n=146), *LRLT* living related liver transplantation (n=220)

During the 1990s, it was shown that the initial poor results were due to the selection of high-risk recipients [15]. The worldwide experience with split liver transplantation reveals that the improvements of patient and graft survival after *ex situ* SLT are more the result of good graft/patient matches and less due to improved techniques (Fig. 3). The realization of this fact led to better patient selection and the procedure became more and more accepted.

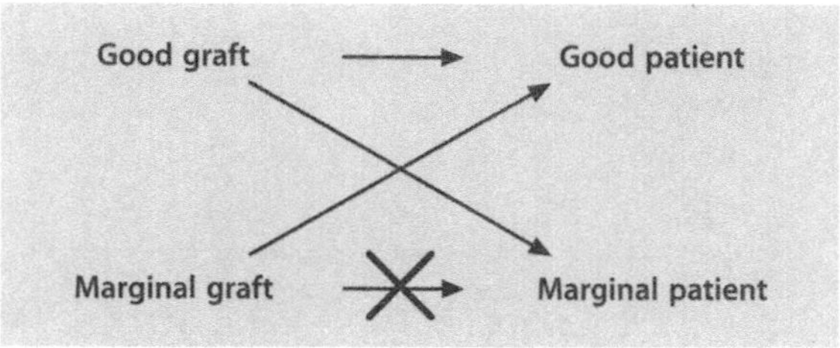

Fig. 3. Graft/patient matching in split liver transplantation

Split liver transplantation (n = 41): 22 left lateral grafts / 19 right lobe grafts
UNOS 1 (high urgent): 4 left lateral SLT (9.75 %)

Patient / Graft survival (median follow up: 12month):

Overall:	90 % / 80 %
Right lobe grafts:	95 % / 95 %
Left lateral grafts:	86 % / 82 %

Complications:

Biliary complications	14.6 %
Vascular complications	4.9 %

Fig. 4. King's College Hospital – single-center experience of 41 split liver transplantations [1]

On the condition of excellent graft/patient matching, single centers like the King's College Hospital London are able to achieve excellent results with *ex situ* split grafts, reaching patient and graft survivals of 90% and 88%, respectively (Fig. 4) [1]. It is their policy to split any good quality organ for one child, requiring emergency or elective liver transplantation and one adult recipient with chronic liver disease [16]. An adult patient requiring emergency transplantation would receive a whole organ and not a part of a liver. These results underline the potential of *ex situ* SLT to achieve similar results as in whole organ transplantation.

The potential of *ex situ* SLT is confirmed by several other groups [1, 11, 13]. Today the patient and graft survival of *ex situ* SLT range between 75–90% and 60–88%, respectively (Table 1).

The experience with *ex situ* SLT in Hamburg (1993–1999) revealed significantly decreased patient and graft survival rates in emergency situations compared to *in situ* split and whole liver transplantation (Fig. 5). The one year patient/graft survival of elective *ex situ* SLT are 76.9%/76.9% and of high urgent *ex situ* SLT 42.9%/35.7%. Based on this experience, *ex situ* split liver grafts are considered second choice grafts in highly urgent situations and should not be used if a whole donor liver is available. This is also very clearly illustrated by the European experience reported by G. de Ville de Goyet [7].

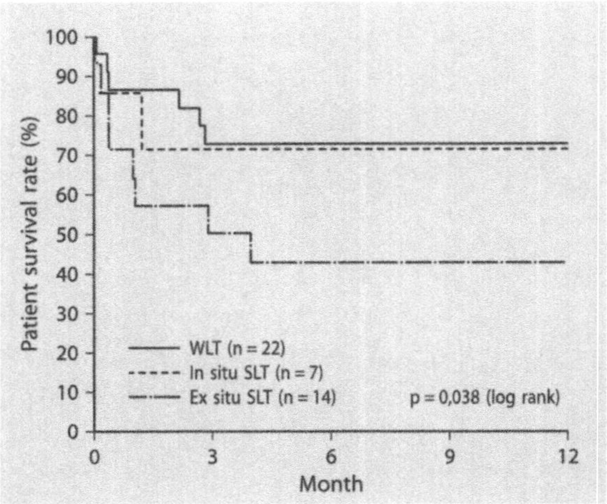

Fig. 5. Patient survival of high urgent split (*ex situ/in situ*) and whole organ liver transplantation (1993–1999). Re-LT are excluded

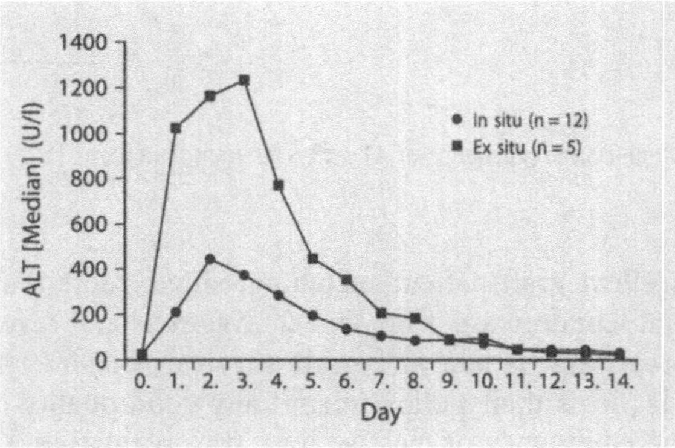

Fig. 6. Postoperative ALT levels. Elective *ex situ* vs *in situ* SLT with similar cold ischemia times (CIT) between 8 and 12 hours. Mean CIT: *ex situ* 561 min (range: 490–715), *in situ* 585 min (range: 505–715)

Ex situ harvested liver grafts sustain more cellular damage during the splitting procedure than *in situ* split grafts, due to the rewarming during backtable splitting. Figure 6 describes the postoperative ALT levels after *ex situ* and *in situ* SLT in elective liver transplantation for chronic liver diseases performed in Hamburg. Despite similar cold ischemia times between 8 and 12 hours, the ALT levels after *ex situ* splitting are much higher during the first few postoperative days in comparison with the *in situ* splitting procedure. Postoperative AST and GLDH levels show a similar pattern to ALT. Additionally to the rewarming injury, the *ex situ* split liver grafts are exposed to significantly prolonged cold ischemia times in contrast to *in situ* harvested split grafts (Fig. 2). At the University Hospital Eppendorf in Hamburg, the mean cold ischemia times in *ex situ* and *in situ* SLT are 723 min and 459 min, respectively.

The above phenomena may explain why *ex situ* SLT does not perform well when patient and graft selection is not strict. In contrast, when excellent grafts are used in elective recipients sufficient reserves are present to obtain excellent results.

Biliary complications have long been recognized as a significant problem in split liver transplantation, affecting 8–25% of recipients (Table 1), with an increased incidence after *ex situ* SLT. The increased incidence of biliary complications in the right lobe graft might be due to excessive dissection of the common bile duct leading to ischemic damage during *ex situ* splitting using the classical technique (Fig. 1). The division of the liver at the line of Cantilie [17] or through the middle of segment IV [18] also leads to a large cut surface and requires the dissection of the hilar plate. Moreover, biliostasis appears more difficult, compared to *in situ* splitting. By using these split techniques, high incidences of biliary complications up to 22% have been reported [7, 18]. The modification of the *ex situ* technique, dividing the liver at the falciform ligament as in *in situ* splitting, leaving the hilar plate untouched, decreased the incidence of biliary complications after *ex situ* splitting considerably [13, 14].

To detect biliary anomalies some authors prefer to perform a cholangiography on the backtable before splitting [18], but it is less common since the modified *ex situ* split technique has been established as the standard technique.

The *ex situ* technique is reported in approximately two thirds of all SLT in the literature. The advantages of *ex situ* splitting are short procurement times and less experienced surgeons can retrieve the organ. Furthermore, fewer resources are needed, which made it more acceptable for the donor hospital.

The comparison between *ex situ* and *in situ* SLT lead to the conclusion that *in situ* SLT is superior to *ex situ* SLT, due to significant shorter ischemia times and no rewarming during liver splitting which led to better initial graft function, increased patient and graft survival, and fewer biliary and vascular complications [13, 19].

As mentioned previously, *ex situ* SLT can achieve results comparable with whole organ liver transplantation or *in situ* SLT, provided that only good quality livers are split and transplanted into stable (elective) patients. Because of the extended ischemic damage, due to the characteristic of the procedure, *ex situ* split liver grafts are not recommendable for emergency transplantation or long distance sharing between transplantation centers. Centers with experience in *ex situ* and *in situ* liver splitting are able to adapt the approach to circumstances. As a consequence, with *in situ* split liver transplantation more risk can be taken with respect to donor quality or recipient status. It is therefore our policy to perform an *in situ* SLT whenever possible. We do accept *ex situ* split liver grafts from excellent donors and for transplantation of elective recipients.

■ Conclusion

Ex situ SLT from cadaveric donors are technical feasible and proved to increase the donor pool for pediatric liver transplantation. Excellent results can be obtained when attention is paid to proper donor and recipient selection as well as clean surgical technique. In the future, it is necessary to define the ideal donor for splitting procedures and to overcome the discretion to share grafts.

■ References

1. Rela M, Vougas V, Muiesan P, Vilca-Melendez H, Smirniotis V, Gibbs P, Karani J, Williams R, Heaton N (1998) Split liver transplantation: King's College Hospital experience. Ann Surg 227(2):282–288
2. Emond JC, Whitington PF, Thistlethwaite JR, Cherqui D, Alonso EA, Woodle IS, Vogelbach P, Busse-Henry SM, Zucker AR, Broelsch CE (1990) Transplantation of two patients with one liver. Analysis of a preliminary experience with 'split-liver' grafting. Ann Surg 212(1):14–22
3. Broelsch CE, Emond JC, Whitington PF, Thistlethwaite JR, Baker AL, Lichtor JL (1990) Application of reduced-size liver transplants as split grafts, auxiliary orthotopic grafts, and living related segmental transplants. Ann Surg 212(3):368–375
4. Otte JB, de Ville de Goyet J, Alberti D, Balladur P, de Hemptinne B (1990) The concept and technique of the split liver in clinical transplantation. Surgery 107(6):605–612
5. Slooff MJ (1995) Reduced size liver transplantation, split liver transplantation, and living related liver transplantation in relation to the donor organ shortage [see comments]. Transpl Int 8:65–68
6. Otte JB (1995) Is it right to develop living related liver transplantation? Do reduced and split livers not suffice to cover the needs? [comment]. Transpl Int 8:69–73
7. De Ville de Goyet J (1995) Split liver transplantation in Europe – 1988 to 1993. Transplantation 59:1371–1376
8. Rogiers X, Malago M, Gawad KA, Kuhlencordt R, Froschle G, Sturm E, Sterneck M, Pothmann W, Schulte am EJ, Burdelski M, Broelsch C (1996) One year of experience with extended application and modified techniques of split liver transplantation. Transplantation 61:1059–1061
9. Kalayoglu M, D'Alessandro AM, Knechtle SJ, Hoffmann RM, Pirsch JD, Judd RH, Armbrust M, Spaith E, Pilli G, Young CJ, Geffner SR, Odorico JS, Sollinger HW, Belzer FO (1996) Preliminary experience with split liver transplantation. J Am Coll Surg 182:381–387
10. Mirza DF, Achilleos O, Pirenne J, Buckels JA, McMaster P, Mayer AD (1998) Encouraging results of split-liver transplantation. Br J Surg 85:494–497
11. Sindhi R, Rosendale J, Mundy D, Taranto S, Baliga P, Reuben A, Rajagopalan PR, Hebra A, Tagge E, Othersen HB Jr (1999) Impact of segmental grafts on pediatric liver transplantation – a review of the United Network for Organ Sharing Scientific Registry data (1990–1996). J Pediatr Surg 34:107–110

12. Chardot C, Branchereau S, de Dreuzy O, Dubuisson C, Pommelet CL, Waguet J, Vellutini G, Gauthier F, Valayer J (1999) Paediatric liver transplantation with a split graft: experience at Bicetre [In Process Citation]. Eur J Pediatr Surg 9:146–152
13. Rogiers X, Topp S, Broering DC (2000) Split Transplantation: split in situ or ex situ? Curr Opin Organ Transplant 5:64–68
14. Reyes J, Gerber D, Mazariegos GV, Casavilla A, Sindhi R, Bueno J, Madariaga J, Fung JJ (2000) Split-liver transplantation: a comparison of ex vivo and in situ techniques. J Pediatr Surg 35(2):283–290
15. Rogiers X, Malago M, Gawad KA, Kuhlencordt R, Fröschle G, Sturm E, et al. (1996) One year of experience with extended application and modified techniques of split liver transplantation. Transplantation 61:1059–1061
16. Rela M, Heaton ND (1998) Split-liver transplantation. Br J Surg 85:881–883
17. Malago M, Rogiers X, Broelsch CE (1997) Liver splitting and living donor techniques. Br Med Bull 53(4):860–867
18. Azoulay D, Astarcioglu I, Bismuth H, Castaing D, et al. (1996) Split-liver transplantation. The Paul Brousse policy. Ann Surg 224(6):737–748
19. Busuttil RW, Goss JA (1999) Split liver transplantation. Ann Surg 229(3):313–321

5.2 Results of *in situ* splitting

R.M. Ghobrial, H. Yersiz, F. Amersi, and R.W. Busuttil

■ Introduction

Orthotopic liver transplantation (OLT) has become a well-established therapeutic modality for patients with end stage liver disease. Improvements in the management of patients, as well as advances in immunosuppression and surgical technique have accounted for remarkable progress in the nearly four decades since the first OLT was performed in 1963 [1, 2]. The full potential for liver replacement is far from being realized because of the widening disparity between rapidly increasing numbers of potential recipients and a severely insufficient cadaveric organ donor supply. Currently, in the United States, it is estimated that more than 15,000 patients are listed for liver transplantation with only 4500 cadaveric livers available annually. With more than 4 million Americans affected with hepatitis C, 25–35% of whom will develop cirrhosis, the transplant community is anticipating an epidemic of patients requiring transplantation. This increasing discrepancy between donor supply and potential recipients has resulted in rising mortality of adult and pediatric patients awaiting OLT.

In order to maximize donor organ utilization in children and adults, four procedures have evolved from the fundamental principle that a portion of the liver with a suitable vascular pedicle, bile duct, and venous drainage along with sufficient functional hepatocyte mass can sustain hepatic function in a patient as well as a whole organ. Reduced-size liver transplantation [3–9] was the wellspring for this effort followed by adult-to-pediatric living-related transplantation [10, 11], cadaveric split liver transplantation [SLT, 12–32] and, more recently, adult-to-adult living-donor transplantation [33].

Since *in situ* split liver transplantation has only been performed over the past four years, there have been only a few published reports with a limited number of patients [29–32, 34]. Initial results from these series suggested an improvement over the *ex vivo* SLT experience, with higher patient and graft survival and lower incidence of complications. However, larger series of *in situ* SLT are required to confirm the results of such initial reports. In addition, a better understanding of the factors that influence the outcome of SLT is critical for the successful application of SLT to expand a severely depleted cadaveric donor pool. This review will outline the outcome of *in situ* SLT and the factors affecting patient survival in our recent series at UCLA that included over 110 *in situ* SLT procedures.

■ Initial *in situ* SLT experience

At UCLA, we first attempted *in situ* split liver transplantation in 1992. Our first experience was not favorable with only one out of four grafts surviving. However, after establishing a living-related liver program and accruing an experience of 30 cases, we resumed the *in situ* split liver program in 1996. In that same year, Rogiers et al. [30] reported their initial experience with 14 split grafts which resulted in a 6 month patient and graft survival rates of 92.8% and 85.7%, respectively (Table 1). Furthermore, the authors described a lower rate of biliary complications, intra-abdominal hemorrhage, and non-function of the right graft as compared with other series utilizing the *ex vivo* split liver techniques. Recently Reyes et al. [34] reported an overall 1-year survival of 96% in 29 patients undergoing *in vivo* SLT. Eight of 29 (27.5%) recipients were high risk. Our initial series at UCLA, which included 28 liver transplants generated from 15 *in situ* splits [31], demonstrated an overall 1-year patient and graft survival of 92.3% and 86%, respectively. In the Hamburg series and the initial UCLA experience, 21.4% and 38.5% of patients, respectively, were urgent recipients.

■ Recent results of *in situ* SLT

Recipient characteristics

All patients listed for liver transplantation were considered as potential candidates for SLT. From July 1996 to December 1999, 102 adult and pediatric (<16 years of age) patients received 110 split liver grafts that included

Table 1. Six month patient and graft survival rates

Series	# Pts	Pt survival	Graft survival	Urgent recipients
Rogiers [30]	14	93%	86%	20%
Goss [31]*	28	92%	86%	36%
Reyes [34]	29	96%	81%	28%
Ghobrial [47]	102	79%	78%	49%

* This series of patients have been included in the series by Ghobrial et al. [47]

54 right trisegments, 53 left lateral segments, one right lobe and two left lobes. Forty-seven right trisegments, one left lobe, one right lobe and one left lateral segment were transplanted into adult recipients. Pediatric patients received fifty-two left lateral segments, seven right trisegments and one left lobe. End stage liver disease caused by biliary atresia was the most common cause of transplantation in pediatric patients, while hepatitis C and fulminant liver failure were the leading causes of transplantation in the adult population.

Candidates for OLT were assigned, according to their medical condition, to one of the following United Network for Organ Sharing (UNOS) categories: UNOS status 1, patients in intensive care with expected survival less than seven days; status 2, continuously hospitalized; and status 3, at home, but requires medical attention. In 1997 UNOS status 1 classification for adult recipients was modified into UNOS status 1 to include fulminant hepatic failure, acute Wilson's disease, primary non-function and hepatic artery thrombosis following OLT; and UNOS status 2A to include patients with chronic liver disease who are in intensive care. Previous UNOS status 2 was changed to 2B. Thus, urgent recipients included UNOS status 1 and 2A. Non-urgent recipients included UNOS status 2, 2B and 3. At the time of SLT, 50 of 102 (49%) recipients were United Network for Organ Sharing, (UNOS) status 1 or 2A and required urgent transplantation. Fifty-two recipients (51%) were non-urgent (UNOS status 2, 2B and 3). Preoperative total serum bilirubin, prothrombin time and serum creatinine ranged from 0.2–37.5 (9.8 ± 9.4) mg/dL, 11–100 (17.5 ± 14.6) seconds, and 0.1–6.6 (0.95 ± 0.9) mg/dL, respectively. Serum aspartate and alanine transaminases (AST and ALT) were 11–17556 (1037 ± 2460) and 9–6170 (664 ± 1240) U/L, respectively. Cold ischemia time ranged between 1.3–10.2 (5.6 ± 2) h with a median of 5.4 hours (h). Median warm ischemia was 35.5 minutes (min) with a mean of 41 ± 19 (17–103) min.

Donor characteristics

All cadaveric livers from donors under 40 years of age were considered for *in situ* splitting. Median donor age was 20 years and median sodium level was 151 mmol/L. Donors with a history of cardiac arrest or hospital stays >5 days were considered for the *in situ* procedure in urgent situations only. Fifteen split liver grafts were obtained from nine donors with a history of cardiac arrest that ranged from 3 to 90 (37.7 ± 28.8) min. Seven grafts originated from four donors with hospital stays that exceeded 5 days. The majority of donors required one pressor to provide hemodynamic stability. Only seventeen grafts were obtained from donors without pressor support. Fifteen grafts were harvested from donors on two pressors and five grafts were obtained from donors on three pressors.

Patient survival

Kaplan-Meier patient survival estimates for all patients who received SLT are shown in Fig. 1. Median follow-up was 14.5 (0–38.7) months. Overall survival rates of patients undergoing SLT at 6 months, 1 and 3 years were 81%, 79%, and 77%, respectively. A matched control cohort of 628 adult and pediatric patients who received a whole organ transplant exhibited overall survival rates of 86%, 82% and 74% at 6 months, 1 and 3 years, respectively (median follow-up time of 16.3 (0–41.9) months, Fig. 1). There was no significant difference in survival between patients who received a SLT when compared to patients transplanted with whole organs (*P* NS). However, among patients who received a SLT, survival of non-urgent recipients (UNOS 2, 2B and 3) was 92%, 89% and 89% at 6 months, 1 and 3 years, respectively (Fig. 2). Survival of urgent (UNOS status 1 and 2A) recipients at 6 months, 1 and 3 years was 70%, 67% and 65%, respectively. Survival of urgent recipients was significantly lower than non-urgent recipients (*P* 0.002, Fig. 2). Figure 3 demonstrates that there was no significant difference in survival of urgent recipients who received a SLT when compared to urgent recipients receiving a whole graft (70%, 67% and 65% ver-

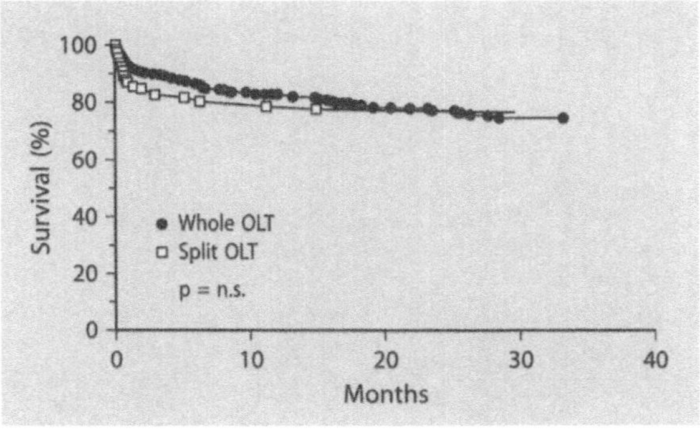

Fig. 1. Overall patient survival following SLT (□) compared to a contemporary cohort of patients who received a whole liver graft (●)

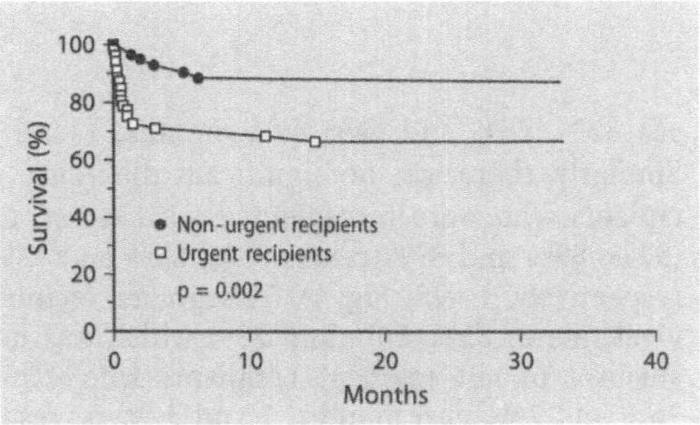

Fig. 2. Kaplan-Meier survival estimates of urgent (UNOS status 1 and 2A, □) compared to non-urgent recipients (UNOS status 2, 2B and 3, ●) of split liver transplantation

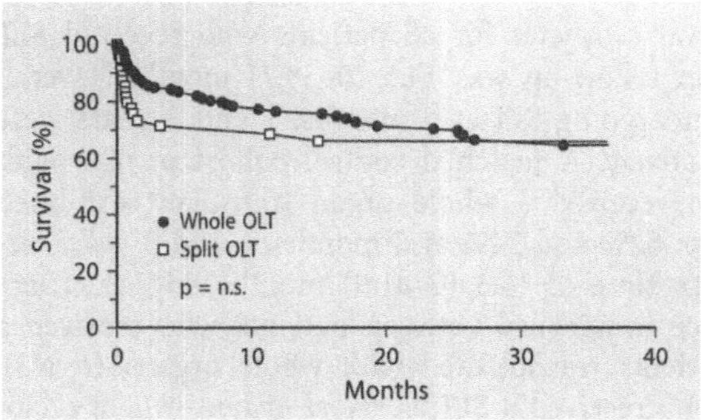

Fig. 3. Survival of urgent (UNOS status 1 and 2A) patients following a split (□) or a whole organ (●) liver transplant

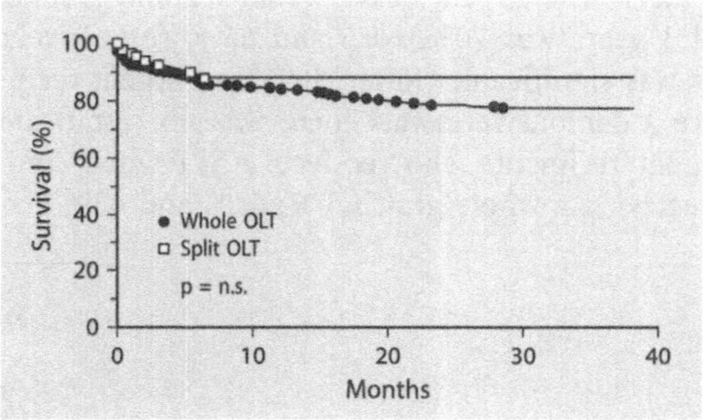

Fig. 4. Survival of non-urgent recipients (UNOS status 2, 2B and 3) following a split (□) or a whole (●) liver transplant

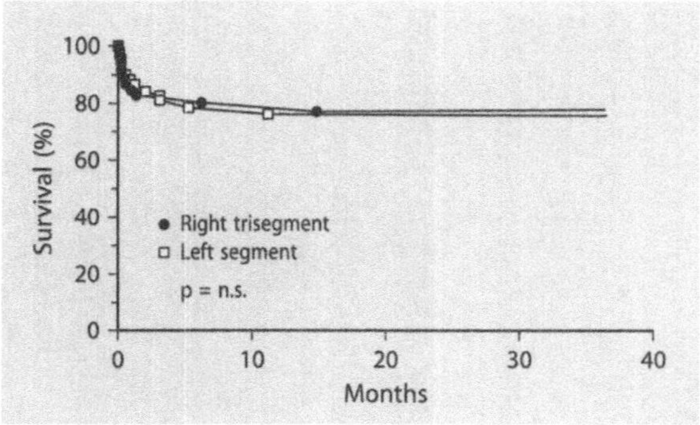

Fig. 5. Patient survival following a right (●) or a left (□) segmental graft

sus 82%, 76% and 64% at 6 months, 1 and 3 years, respectively; *P* NS). Similarly, there was no significant difference in survival of non-urgent recipients who were transplanted with either a split or a whole organ graft (92%, 89% and 89% versus 89%, 85% and 78% at 6 months, 1 and 3 years, respectively, *P* NS; Fig. 4). Trisegment recipients exhibited an overall survival rate of 83%, 80% and 78% which was not significantly different from survival of left segment recipients who exhibited survival rates of 78%, 76% and 76% at 6 months, 1 and 3 years, respectively (*P* NS, Fig. 5).

Although our overall patient survival of 81%, 79% and 77% at 6 months, 1 and 3 years, respectively, is lower than previous reports using this procedure; our recent experience with SLT included an extremely high number of high-risk patients. At the time of transplantation, 49% of the patients were high-risk (UNOS status 1 and 2A) recipients. When patients were stratified according to UNOS status, survival of non-urgent recipients was superior to that of high-risk recipients after SLT. In addition, among urgent high-risk recipients, survival of patients who received a SLT was not significantly different from those who received a whole organ. Similarly, survival of non-urgent recipients was similar whether a split or a whole organ was utilized. Thus, *in situ* SLT affords patient survival rates that are equivalent to whole organ transplantation.

Causes of death after SLT

Ten children and 13 adult patients died after SLT. Eighteen (36%) deaths were encountered in 50 urgent (UNOS status 1, 2A) recipients. In contrast, only 5 deaths occurred in 52 non-urgent (UNOS status 2 and 3, 9.6%) patients after SLT. Sepsis was the leading cause of death in urgent recipients resulting in seven of the eighteen deaths (41%). Graft failure was the underlying cause of death in only 4 urgent patients. In contrast, three of five deaths in non-urgent recipients were caused by graft failure. Only 3 late deaths occurred after SLT at 161, 341 and 453 days and were caused by multi-organ failure in one and sepsis in two patients. Twenty of 23 deaths (87%) occurred within the first 100 days after OLT. Thus sepsis, but not graft failure, was the leading cause of death after SLT.

The causes of death after SLT are similar to what has been reported following whole organ transplantation. In patients who underwent OLT for HCV at our institution, sepsis was the cause of death in 37.8% of patients who died after whole organ OLT [35]. Similarly, 26% of deaths in patients undergoing transplantation for primary sclerosing cholangitis were related to sepsis [36]. A high incidence of death due to sepsis in the late postoperative period has also been reported after whole organ transplantation [37, 38].

Predictors of patient survival after SLT

Since splitting of the liver may have contributed to recipient deaths within 100 of transplantation, factors that may influence patient survival during this period were subjected to further analysis. Recipient variables examined were age, weight, UNOS status prior to transplantation, number of transplants per patient, pretransplant mechanical ventilation, preoperative bilirubin, prothrombin time, serum creatinine, and type of split liver graft type. The eight donor variables that were considered included donor age, sodium level, days of hospitalization prior to procurement, history of cardiac arrest, donor serum bilirubin, AST, ALT, and number of donor pressors. In addition, two operative variables that included cold and warm ischemia times were analyzed.

By univariate comparison, two variables were significantly associated with patient survival following SLT. Such variables included UNOS status of the patient (urgent UNOS status 1 and 2A versus non-urgent UNOS 2, 2B and 3; *P* 0.002) and number of transplants per patient (2 versus 1, *P* 0.003). Preoperative recipient mechanical ventilation (*P* 0.091), preoperative prothrombin time (>11.3, *P* 0.187), donor sodium level (>150 mmol/L, *P* 0.132), donor length of hospital stay (>5 days, *P* 0.069), and operative warm ischemia time (>35.5 min, *P* 0.077) all approached statistical significance. Neither the type of graft utilized (right trisegment versus left lateral segment, *P* 0.835; NS), nor the age of the recipient (>16 versus <16 versus >16 years, *P* 0.268; NS) influenced patient survival after SLT. All variables were subjected to multivariate logistic regression analysis. Of these, one recipient and one donor variable were identified as independent predictors of survival: UNOS status of the recipient (urgent versus non-urgent, *P* 0.003) and donor hospital stay (>5 days, *P* 0.063) with relative risk factors of 7.2 and 1, respectively.

Thus, univariate analysis of recipient, donor and operative factors identified two significant variables that adversely affect patient survival following SLT. Such variables included a high recipient UNOS status (1 and 2A) and requirement for retransplantation (2 versus 1 transplants). Preoperative mechanical ventilation and elevated prothrombin time were two other recipient variables that approached, but did not reach, statistical significance. All such variables, particularly an advanced UNOS status, were identified by multiple other studies as predictors of poor patient survival following whole organ OLT [39, 40]. Age group, number of transplants and UNOS status were identified as independent risk factors for patient death in a study that evaluated 250 patients who underwent retransplantation at UCLA [41]. Other variables that approached statistical significance on univariate analysis after SLT included donor sodium level (>150 mmol/L), donor length of hospital stay (>5 days), and operative warm ischemia time (>35.5 min). A large study that analyzed 340 whole OLTs demonstrated that donor plasma sodium >155 mmol/L and AB0 incompatibility were independent predictors for patient and graft survival [42]. The deleterious effects of prolonged warm ischemia time on the outcome of whole organ transplantation is well established [40, 43]. Similarly, prolonged donor hospitalization has been clearly demonstrated to adversely effect graft and patient survival after whole organ grafts [40, 44, 45]. In addition, multivariate analysis identified donor hospital stay (>5 days) and the UNOS status of recipients as independent predictors of survival following SLT. In contrast to other published reports, our study did not demonstrate that the age of the recipient [41, 46] or the type of graft used (right versus left) adversely affected patient survival [4, 14]. It therefore appears that factors affecting patient survival after SLT are similar to those previously identified for whole organ transplantation.

■ Conclusions

During the last four years we have extensively used the *in situ* split procedure to maximize the utilization of our cadaveric pool for both adult and pediatric patients. Despite the intuitive appeal of SLT as an innovative approach for the scarcity of liver donors, poor initial results with reduced-size and *ex vivo* split grafts have resulted in slow acceptance of the procedure. In recent years, national debate on organ allocation has underscored the acute need for a renewed interest in SLT. Our recent results clearly indicate that the outcome of *in situ* SLT is equivalent to that achieved by whole organ transplantation. We have therefore pursued an aggressive policy to split suitable livers into right trisegmental and left lateral grafts to maximally benefit both the adult and pediatric populations [28]. We are currently pursuing the option of a right and a left lobe split that would benefit two appropriately size-matched adult recipients. We have also developed institutional donor, operative and recipient criteria for SLT. Hemodynamically stable cadaveric donors under the age of 45 years are considered for the split procedure if the liver is deemed suitable by the harvesting team. We avoid the utilization of donors who exhibit sodium levels >155 mmol/L, hospital stays >5 days, a history of cardiac arrest, or on more than one pressor except in extremely desperate circumstances. Cold ischemia time is ideally kept below 6 hours and transplantation of split grafts with cold ischemia times >10 hours should be avoided. Warm ischemia time should not exceed 45 min. With the current organ allocation system that favors urgent recipients it is practically impossible to avoid transplantation of split organs in UNOS status 1 or 2A recipients. Moreover, splitting a liver graft for an urgent recipient is likely to benefit another non-urgent patient. Such insight is validated by our current results that demonstrate equal survival rates of high-risk patients whether they received a split or a whole organ graft.

In summary, *in situ* SLT is performed in non-urgent recipient with excellent results. Despite a lower patient survival in high-risk recipients, SLT can be applied to the urgent patient with results that are equivalent to those expected with whole organs. Independent variables adversely affecting patient survival after SLT include donor hospital stay >5 days and high-risk urgent patients. Other factors that may impact patient survival include retransplantation, preoperative mechanical ventilation, elevated prothrombin time, donor sodium level and prolonged warm ischemia. SLT should be applied to expand the donor organ pool and benefit a larger number of patients.

References

1. Starzl TE, Marchiaro TL, Von Kaulla K, et al. (1963) Homotransplantation of the liver in humans. Surg Gynecol Obstet 117:659–676
2. NIH Consensus Development Conference Statement (1983) Liver transplantation. June 20–23 Hepatology 4:1075
3. Bismuth H, Houssin D (1984) Reduced-sized orthotopic liver graft in hepatic transplantation in children. Surgery 95:367–370
4. Broelsch CE, Emond JC, Thistlethwaite JR, et al. (1988) Liver transplantation, including the concept of reduced-size liver transplants in children. Ann Surg 208:410–420
5. Broelsch CE, Emond JC, Whitington PF, et al. (1990) Application of reduced size liver transplants as split grafts, auxiliary orthotopic grafts and living related segmental transplants. Ann Surg 214:368–370
6. Emond JC, Whitington PF, Thistlethwaite JR, et al. (1989) Reduced-size orthotopic liver transplantation: use in the management of children with chronic liver disease. Transplantation 10:867–872
7. Houssin D, Soubrane O, Boillot O, et al. (1992) Orthotopic liver transplantation with a reduced-size graft: an ideal compromise in pediatrics? Surgery 111:532–542
8. Langnas AN, Wagner CM, Inagaki M, et al. (1992) The results of reduced-size liver transplantation, including split livers, in patients with end-stage liver disease. Transplantation 53:387–391
9. Otte JB, de Ville de Goyet J, Solak E, et al. (1990) Size reduction of the donor liver is a safe way to alleviate the shortage of size-matched organs in pediatric liver transplantation. Ann Surg 211:146–157
10. Raia S, Nery JR, Mies S (1988) Liver transplantation from live donors. Lancet 2:497
11. Strong RW, Lynch SV, Ong TN, et al. (1990) Successful liver transplantation from a living donor to her son. N Eng J Med 322:1505–1507
12. Pichlmayr R, Ringe B, Gubernatis G, et al. (1988) Transplantation einer Spenderleber auf zwei Empfänger (splitting – transplantation): eine neue Methode in der Weiterentwicklung der Lebersegmenttransplantation. Langenbecks Arch Chir 373:127–130
13. Bismuth H, Marino M, Castaing D (1989) Emergency orthotopic liver transplantation in two patients using one donor. Br J Surg 76:722–724
14. Azoulay D, Astarcioglu I, Bismuth H, et al. (1996) Split liver transplantation: The Paul Brousse policy. Ann Surg 224:737–748
15. Broelsch CE, Emond JC, Whitington PF, et al. (1990) Application of reduced size liver transplants as split grafts, auxiliary orthotopic grafts and living related segmental transplants. Ann Surg 214:368–377
16. De Ville de Goyet J (1995) Split liver transplantation in Europe, 1988–1993. Transplantation 59:1371–1376
17. Emond JC, Whitington PF, Thistlethwaite JR, et al. (1990) Transplantation of two patients with one liver. Analysis of a preliminary experience with 'split-liver' grafting. Ann Surg 212:14–22
18. Houssin D, Boillot O, Soubrane O, et al. (1993) Controlled liver splitting for transplantation in two recipients: technique, results and perspectives. Br J Surg 80:75–80

19. Kalayoglu M, D'Alessandro AM, Knechtle JS, et al. (1996) Preliminary experience with split liver transplantation. J Am Col Surg 182:381–387
20. Langnas AN, Wagner CM, Inagaki M, et al. (1992) The results of reduced-size liver transplantation, including split livers, in patients with end-stage liver disease. Transplantation 53:387–391
21. Mirza DF, Achilleos O, Pirenne J, et al. (1998) Encouraging results of split-liver transplantation. Br J Surg 85:494–497
22. Otte JB (1995) Is it right to develop living related liver transplantation? Do reduced and split livers not suffice to cover the needs? Transpl Int 8:69–73
23. Otte JB, de Ville de Goyet J, Alberti D, et al. (1990) The concept and technique of the split liver in clinical transplantation. Surgery 107:605–612
24. Rela M, Voregas V, Miniesan P, et al. (1998) Split liver transplantation: King's College Hospital experience. Ann Surg 227:282–288
25. Rogiers X, Malago M, Gawad KA, et al. (1996) One year experience with extended application and modified techniques of split liver transplantation. Transplantation 61:1059–1061
26. Sloof MJH (1995) Reduced size liver transplantation, split liver transplantation and living related transplantation in relation to donor organ shortage. Transpl Int 8:65–68
27. Reyes J, Gerber D, Mazariegos GV, et al. (2000) Split-liver transplantation: a comparison of ex vivo and in situ techniques. J Ped Surg 35:283–290
28. Busuttil RW, Goss JA (1999) Split liver transplantation. Ann Surg 229(3):313–321
29. Rogiers X, Malago M, Habib N, et al. (1995) *In situ* splitting of the liver in heart-beating cadaveric organ donor for transplantation in two recipients. Transplantation 59:1081–1083
30. Rogiers X, Malago M, Gawad K, et al. (1996) *In situ* splitting of cadaveric livers: the ultimate expansion of the donor pool. Ann Surg 224:331–341
31. Goss JA, Yersiz H, Shackleton CR, et al. (1997) In situ splitting of the cadaveric liver for transplantation. Transplantation 64:871–877
32. Ghobrial RM, Farmer DG, Yersiz H, et al. (1998) Split liver transplantation for expansion of the donor pool. Transplantation 67(9):S548
33. Marcos A, Fisher R, Ham J, et al. (1999) Right lobe living donor liver transplantation. Transplantation 68(6):798–803
34. Reyes J, Gerber D, Mazariegos GV, et al. (2000) Split-liver transplantation: a comparison of ex-vivo and in situ techniques. J Ped Surg 35:283–290
35. Ghobrial RM, Farmer DG, Baquerizo A, et al. (1999) Orthotopic liver transplantation for hepatitis C: outcome, effect of immunosuppression and causes of retransplantation during an eight year single center experience. Ann Surg 229(6):824–831
36. Graziadel IW, Wiesner RH, Marotta PJ, et al. (1999) Long-term results of patients undergoing liver transplantation for primary sclerosing cholangitis. Hepatology 30:1121–1127
37. Asfar S, Metrakos P, Fryer J, et al. (1996) An analysis of late deaths after liver transplantation. Transplantation 61:1377–1381
38. Ryckman FC, Alonso MH, Bucuvalas JC, Balistreri WF (1999) Long-term survival after liver transplantation. J Ped Surg 34:845–850
39. Wong T, Devlin J, Roland N, Heaton, Williams R (1997) Clinical characteristics affecting the outcome of liver retransplantation. Transplantation 64:878–882

40. Strasberg SM, Howard TK, Molmenti EP, Hertl M (1994) Selecting the donor liver: risk factors for poor function after orthotopic liver transplantation. Hepatology 20:829–838
41. Markmann JF, Markowitz JS, Yersiz H, et al. (1997) Long-term survival after retransplantation of the liver. Ann Surg 226:408–420
42. Figuras J, Busquets J, Grande L, et al. (1996) The deleterious effect of donor high plasma sodium and extended preservation in liver transplantation. A multivariate analysis. Transplantation 61:410–413
43. Mimeault R, Grant D, Ghent C, Duff J, Wall W (1989) Analysis of donor and recipient variables and early graft function after orthotopic liver transplantation. Transplant Proc 21(2):3355
44. Mor E, Klintmalm GB, Gonwa TA, et al. (1992) The use of marginal donors for liver transplantation. Transplant Proc 53:383–386
45. Ploeg RJ, D'Alessandro AM, Knechtle SJ, et al. (1993) Risk factors for primary dysfunction after liver transplantation: a multivariate analysis. Transplantation 55:807–813
46. Cacciarelli TV, Esquivel CO, Moore DH, et al. (1997) Factors affecting survival after orthotopic liver transplantation in infants. Transplantation 64 (2):242–248
47. Ghobrial RM, Yersiz H, Farmer D, et al. (2000) Predictors of survival after in situ split liver transplantation: analysis of 110 consecutive cases. Ann Surg 232:312–323

5.3

M.J.H. Slooff and E. Sieders

The paradigm of split liver transplantation: a word of caution

■ Introduction

The first reports on split liver transplantation in the early 1980s gave rise to great expectations because it became clear that splitting a graft for two recipients was technically feasible [1, 2]. As a consequence, the shortage of donors for pediatric patients could be alleviated without detrimental effects on the pool for adult recipients [3]. Therefore, one should expect that a technique which increases the number of grafts for transplantation and thereby reduces waiting list time and mortality, especially in the field of pediatric transplantation, should have become a popular method of transplantation. However, the percentage of split liver transplantations of the total number of performed transplantations hardly increased in the following years. When analyzing data from the UNOS registry, split liver transplantation made up only about 5% of all performed pediatric liver transplantations in 1996 [4]. In 1999, data of Eurotransplant International and of the European Liver Transplant Registry showed that split liver transplantation made up between 4 and 9% of all performed liver transplantations [5, 6]. It is obvious that despite the practical and theoretical advantages of splitting livers, there seems still to be some restraint for using this technique in the majority of liver transplant centers. However, split liver transplantation is not only a necessity but it also deserves broader application because the results can be improved if certain precautions are taken. By analyzing a single center's experience, this chapter aims at indicating some crucial factors for a successful split liver program.

■ Split liver transplantation – the Groningen experience

Between 1990 and 1999, 27 split liver transplantations were performed in the University Hospital Groningen (the Netherlands) of which 14 were transplanted simultaneously. Eighteen split transplantations were performed in 16 children and nine were performed in adult patients. Two children, who received a split liver graft in a primary transplantation, also un-

Table 1. Patient and graft survival in the period 1990–1999

		1-month	6-months	1-year	P-value
Patient survival					
Children	Split liver transplantation (16)	88% (14)	88% (13)	74% (10)	
	Reduced-size liver transplantation [1] (47)	72% (34)	72% (34)	70% (30)	0.84 [2]
	Full size liver transplantation [1] (47)	96% (45)	96% (40)	96% (37)	0.06 [2]
Adults	Split liver transplantation (9)	73% (7)	53% (4)	53% (4)	
	Full size transplantation [1] (271)	92% (249)	86% (222)	84% (206)	0.11 [3]
Graft survival					
Children	Split liver transplantation (18)	61% (11)	56% (10)	44% (8)	
	Reduced-size liver transplantation (72)	67% (48)	67% (46)	64% (40)	0.18 [2]
	Full size liver transplantation (55)	76% (42)	74% (36)	72% (32)	0.02 [2]
Adults	Split liver transplantation (9)	56% (5)	42% (3)	42% (3)	
	Full size transplantation (307)	88% (271)	80% (234)	77% (213)	0.05 [3]

[1] Graft type based on primary transplantation. Patients never had a split liver graft
[2] P-value versus children with split liver transplantation
[3] P-value versus adults with split liver transplantation

derwent a retransplantation with a split liver graft. Twenty-four liver grafts were procured with the *ex situ* technique and the remaining three grafts with *in situ* technique. In 11 transplantations a segmental graft consisting of segments II and III was used. Of 10 right liver lobe grafts consisting of segments V–VIII, one graft also included segment IV and one also included segment I. Of six left liver lobe grafts consisting of segments II–IV, one included segment I as well.

Actuarial patient and graft survival rates after split liver transplantation are listed in Table 1.

When analyzing surgical complications after split liver transplantation, seven transplants were complicated by a vascular complication: three grafts (11%) were complicated by hepatic artery thrombosis, two (7%) by portal vein thrombosis, one (4%) by combined hepatic artery and portal vein thrombosis, and one (4%) by torsion of the inferior caval vein. Six transplants (23%) were complicated by biliary complications. The main biliary complication was the occurrence of a biloma due to bile leakage from the resection surface. This occurred two times after liver lobe grafting and three times after segmental grafting. In one case a biloma was accompanied by stenosis of the bile duct and in one case by ischemic type biliary structures. A sixth graft was complicated by bile duct stenosis. Postoperative bleeding complications which required one or more surgical interven-

Table 2. Absolute timetable of eight split liver procedures in hours

	D1	D2	D3	D4	D5	D6	D7	D8
Start CIT – start split procedure	5	5.5	7	6.5	6.3	11.5	3.5	9.2
Start – end split procedure	4	3.5	4	3.5	3.5	2	3	3.8
End split procedure – start SLT	0.5	0.5	1	3	0.7	0	0.5	0.5
	0.5	0.5	S	S	0	0	S	S
Start SLT – start reperfusion	3	5	3.5	6	4.3	3.5	3.5	3.5
	3	7.5	S	S	6.7	4	S	S
Total CIT	12.5	14.5	15.5	19	14.8	17	10.5	17
	12.5	17	S	S	16.5	17.5	S	S

D donor; *CIT* cold ischemia time; *SLT* split liver transplantation; *S* shared graft

tions occurred after six transplantations (23%): in five cases after right liver lobe grafting and in one case after left lobe grafting. These bleeding complications were the indications for in total 13 surgical interventions and contributed to the loss of three grafts. Overall, 38 surgical interventions had to be performed, including 8 retransplantations (30%).

In this series, survival rates after split liver transplantation are disappointing and morbidity was high. Therefore, to understand these results, characteristics of recipients, donors and transplantation procedures were analyzed in more detail. Two issues emerged from this analysis. First, a considerable number of patients (n=11, 44%) who received a split liver graft were transplanted urgently (Eurotransplant International code high urgency or UNOS code I or II) and 14 (56%) patients were transplanted electively. Of the urgently transplanted patients only 5 (46%) survived compared with 11 (79%) of the electively transplanted patients. A second striking issue was an overall median cold ischemia time of 13 hours (range 6–18 hours). When comparing six grafts with a cold ischemia time shorter than 10 hours with 21 grafts with a cold ischemia time longer than 10 hours, three grafts (50%) of the first group survived and only seven (33%) of the latter group. To provide insight into the origin of such a long cold ischemia time and thereby into the logistics of a split procedure, timetables of the first eight split liver procedures were analyzed (Table 2). These data revealed that between the start of the cold ischemia time in the donor and the start of the split procedure, 41% of the cold ischemia time was lost and that the split procedure itself consumed 23% of the total cold ischemia time.

■ Discussion

The restraint for splitting livers mainly originates from disappointing results in terms of low patient and graft survival and a high morbidity rate as reported in the present series as well as by other early series [7, 8]. After analysis of our limited experience we found two factors determining the outcome. Patients needing a graft on an urgent basis should not receive a split liver graft. This fact is supported by the experience of other centers as shown in Table 3. A careful patient selection will therefore have a positive influence on the outcome after split liver transplantation and may subsequently improve its dissemination among the transplant centers. Furthermore, logistics are important. Cold ischemia times were too long in our series. Transport of shared grafts between distant centers was one contributing factor. Also, too much time elapsed between the arrival of the organ and the start of the split procedure itself. It became clear, also from our recent experience, that the cold ischemia time should be kept as short as possible to improve the outcome. By making use of the *in situ* split technique, cold ischemia times will decrease [9]. However, this technique requires longer operation times in donor hospitals, a fact which will not always be appreciated by these hospitals. Morbidity comprising vascular, biliary, and postoperative bleeding complications is not exclusively associated with the split technique. Such complications do also occur after transplantation of full size and reduced-size grafts [10, 11].

Not only technical and logistical factors play a role in the further dissemination of split liver transplantation, but administrative barriers to perform split liver transplantation in a selected patient category with carefully selected donor organs should also be removed, for example by composing an exclusive dual-recipient split liver waiting list as proposed by Strasberg et al. [12]. To establish such a program, an expansion of split liver transplant centers and collaboration between these centers is required. An additional advantage will be the shortening of the cold ischemia time with consequently fewer postoperative complications.

Table 3. Reports on *ex situ* split liver transplantation based on the proportion of high urgency patients

Author	High urgency (%)	Patient survival (%)	Graft survival (%)
Broelsch [7]	40	60	43
Shaw [13]	70	50	50
Houssin [14]	56	75	69
de Ville [15]	33	68	62
Azoulay [16]	7	81	78
Kalayoglu [17]	8	91	75
Rela [18]	12	90	88

A matter seldom discussed is the fact that bipartitioning of the liver requires considerable skill, anatomical knowledge, and experience in the field of liver surgery. These are probably major reasons why so many centers are reluctant toward this procedure. The centers active in split liver transplantation, at least in Europe, are mostly performing liver transplantations in the frame work of hepatobiliary surgery.

In conclusion, the restraint for splitting livers was initially justified. However, new insights have been gained which improves the outcome after split liver transplantation. Therefore, the technique deserves wider application.

■ References

1. Pichlmayr R, Ringe B, Gubernatis G, Hauss J, Bunzendahl H (1988) Transplantation einer Spenderleber auf zwei Empfänger (Splitting-Transplantation): Eine neue Methode in der Weiterentwicklung der Lebersegmenttransplantation. Langenbecks Arch Chir 373:127–130
2. Emond JC, Whitington PF, Thistlethwaite JR, et al. (1990) Transplantation of two patients with one liver. Analysis of a preliminary experience with 'split-liver' grafting. Ann Surg 212:14–22
3. Slooff MJ (1995) Reduced size liver transplantation, split liver transplantation, and living related liver transplantation in relation to the donor organ shortage. Transpl Int 8:65–68
4. Sindhi R, Rosendale J, Mundy D, et al. (1999) Impact of segmental grafts on pediatric liver transplantation – a review of the United Network for Organ Sharing Scientific Registry data (1990–1996). J Pediatr Surg 34:107–110
5. Persijn G (2000) Eurotransplant International Foundation. Personal communication
6. Adam R, Bismuth H, Castaing D, Bustany P, Karam V, Cailliez V (1999) Registry of the European Liver Transplant Association; Data Analysis 05/1968–12/1997. Hpital Paul Brousse Villejuf, France
7. Broelsch CE, Emond JC, Whitington PF, Thistlethwaite JR, Baker AL, Lichtor JL (1990) Application of reduced-size liver transplants as split grafts, auxiliary orthotopic grafts, and living related segmental transplants. Ann Surg 212:368–375
8. Shaw BW Jr, Wood RP, Stratta RJ, et al. (1990) Management of arterial anomalies encountered in split-liver transplantation. Transplant Proc 22:420–422
9. Rogiers X, Malago M, Gawad K, et al. (1996) In situ splitting of cadaveric livers: the ultimate expansion of a limited donor pool. Ann Surg 224:331–339
10. De Ville de Goyet J, Hausleithner V, Reding R, Lerut J, Janssen M, Otte JB (1993) Impact of innovative techniques on the waiting list and results in pediatric liver transplantation. Transplantation 56:1130–1136
11. Sieders E, Peeters PM, TenVergert EM, et al. (1999) Analysis of survival and morbidity after pediatric liver transplantation with full-size and technical-variant grafts. Transplantation 68:540–545
12. Strasberg SM, Lowell JA, Howard TK (1999) Reducing the shortage of donor livers: what would it take to reliably split livers for transplantation into two adult recipients? Liver Transpl Surg 5:437–450

13. Shaw BW Jr, Wood RP, Stratta RJ, et al. (1990) Management of arterial anomalies encountered in split-liver transplantation. Transplant Proc 22:420–422
14. Houssin D, Boillot O, Soubrane O, et al. (1993) Controlled liver splitting for transplantation in two recipients: technique, results and perspectives. Br J Surg 80:75–80
15. De Ville de Goyet J (1995) Split liver transplantation in Europe – 1988 to 1993. Transplantation 59:1371–1376
16. Azoulay D, Astarcioglu I, Bismuth H, et al. (1996) Split-liver transplantation. The Paul Brousse policy. Ann Surg 224:737–746
17. Kalayoglu M, D'Alessandro AM, Knechtle SJ, et al. (1996) Preliminary experience with split liver transplantation. J Am Coll Surg 182:381–387
18. Rela M, Vougas V, Muiesan P, et al. (1998) Split liver transplantation: King's College Hospital experience. Ann Surg 227:282–288

5.4

D. Azoulay, G. Marin-Hargreaves, and H. Bismuth

Split liver transplant for two adults: initial experience at Paul Brousse Hospital

■ Introduction

The feasibility of splitting the liver prior to transplantation depends on the surgical application of the anatomical segmentation of the liver, as described by Couinaud [1]. The technique was first described by Pichlmayr in 1988 [2] in an adult and a child. Extending its use together with that of liver reduction techniques (in which a large volume of healthy liver may be discarded) [3], and increasing experience have considerably reduced the number of children awaiting liver transplantation [4]. However, the number of patients waiting for a liver to be transplanted increases as new indications are added and makes the scarcity of available organs more and more serious; with adult potential recipients accounting for >95% of the waiting-list deaths [5].

In 1989, Bismuth was the first to perform liver transplantation to two adult patients from one donor liver, to cope with the emergency due to two cases of fulminant hepatitis requiring transplantation at the same time [6]. From that episode, the experience gained from extensive use of split livers for an adult and a child at the same time and also the recently developed programs of living-related liver donation, in order to increase the pool of grafts for our recipients, we have evolved the policy of, whenever feasible, systematically splitting liver grafts. We do this by using *ex situ* splitting of cadaver donors and *in situ* splitting of livers from patients with familial amyloidotic polyneuropathy undergoing domino liver transplantation [7].

■ The Paul Brousse experience

From July 1993 to December 1999, 34 adults had split liver transplantation using grafts obtained from optimal donors [8] (age under 55 years old, body weight over 70 kg, stable hemodynamics, normal function tests, and no macroscopic aspect of liver steatosis at harvesting [9]). The technical aspects of the procedure have been described in another chapter. However we stress the importance of the adaptability of the cutting line since in the last 6 cases of splitting the liver, segment IV of Couinaud [1] was included in the left graft, thus, increasing the graft to recipient body weight ratio (GBWR) for this side. In the previous cases, the middle hepatic vein was kept with the right graft as the liver was divided through the middle of segment IV.

Grafts were prepared by *ex situ* split in 30 cases or by *in situ* split in 4 cases. In the latter, although the operating time in the donor is longer, better hemostasis is achieved and fewer biliary complications have been reported [8, 10].

Morbidity

The complication rate was 24% overall, with 6% being arterial complications. Biliary complications were recorded in 22% of the cases, and were related either to leaks from the raw surface or to problems with the biliary anastomosis, particularly stenosis. A wider use of microsurgical techniques should improve technique-related morbidity.

Survival

Overall patient survival at 2 years was similar for patients whether they had received a whole liver, or a right or left split liver: 85%, 74% and 64%, respectively. This was due to three retransplantations in the recipients of a left split graft after primary non-function (PNF).

Patient survival after split liver transplantation in the Paul Brousse series has been found to be influenced by graft steatosis and hospitalization of the recipient. Factors influencing graft survival are graft steatosis and GBWR < 1%.

■ Coordination and logistical aspects

Several aspects have to be taken into consideration. The importance of the number of operations performed by the team has been well established in liver transplantation [11], and the same applies for split liver transplantation (SLT), since better results have been reported from centers that have performed more than 40 SLT [12].

Coordination between transplantation centers acquainted with the technique should optimize the use of split grafts, when two surgical teams or two optimal recipients are not readily available in one center alone. Moreover, a pool of size-matched patients particularly of left split liver grafts may, therefore, be made available.

Finally, *in situ* splitting requires agreement with donor hospitals and other procurement teams, since the operating time in the donor is prolonged by 2 to 3 hours.

■ Conclusion

From our experience, split liver transplantation for two adults is a real possibility to help overcome organ shortage. It appears to be necessary to obtain an adequate mass of functional parenchyma (over 1% of the graft-body weight ratio), particularly for the left split graft recipients, as already shown in whole liver transplantation [13]. Minimal dissection on the hilar plate to avoid biliary devascularization, and shortening the cold ischemia time through *in situ* splitting – whenever practicable – should be principles rather than objectives when aiming at splitting the liver for transplantation.

Furthermore, a strict selection criteria of optimal recipients for split-liver grafts and precise allocation to size- and sex-matched recipients are aspects which still require attention.

The increasing experience of liver transplantation centers with splitting techniques has improved results in recent years. A similar evolution is to be expected in split liver transplantation for two adults, and this should have a considerable effect in expanding the available pool of donors for adult patients, with results comparable to those of whole liver transplantation [8].

■ References

1. Couinaud C (1957) Le foie. Etudes anatomiques et chirurgicales. Masson, Paris
2. Pichlmayr R, Ringe B, Gubernatis G, Hauss J, Bunzendahl H (1988) Transplantation einer Spenderleber auf zwei Empfänger (Split liver transplantation). Eine neue Methode in der Weiterentwicklung der Lebersegment Transplantation. Langenbecks Archiv für Chirurgie 373:127–130
3. Bismuth H, Houssin D (1984) Reduced-size orthotopic liver graft in hepatic transplantation in children. Surgery 95:367–370
4. Busuttil RW, Goss JA (1999) Split liver transplantation. Review. Ann Surg 229:313–321
5. Smith CME (1977) Annual Report of the US Scientific Registry of Transplant Recipients and the Organ Procurement and Transplantation Network – Transplant Data: 1988–1996. UNOS, Richmond, VA, and the Division of Transplantation, Bureau of Health Resources and Services Administration, US Department of Health and Human Services, Rockville, MD
6. Bismuth H, Morino M, Castaing D, et al. (1989) Emergency orthotopic liver transplantation in two patients using one donor liver. Br J Surg 76:722–724

7. Azoulay D, Castaing D, Adam R, et al. (2000) Transplantation of three adult patients with one cadaveric graft: wait or innovate. Liver Transplant Surg 6:239–240
8. Azoulay D, Castaing D, Adam R, et al. (2001) Split liver transplantation for two adult recipients: feasibility and long term outcomes. Ann Surg 233(4):565–574
9. Azoulay D, Astarcioglu I, Bismuth H, et al. (1996) Split-liver transplantation: The Paul Brousse policy. Ann Surg 224:737–748
10. Rogiers X, Malago M, Gawad K, et al. (1996) In situ splitting of cadaveric livers: the ultimate expansion of the donor pool. Ann Surg 224:331–341
11. Edwards EB, Roberts JP, McBride MA, et al. (1999) The effect of the volume of procedures at transplantation centers on mortality after liver transplantation. N Engl J Med 341:2049–2053
12. European Transplant Registry (1999) Data analysis 05/1968–06/1999. ELTR, Villejuif
13. Adam R, Castaing D, Bismuth H (1993) Transplantation of small donor livers in adult recipients. Transplant Proc 25:1105–1106

5.5 H. Bismuth

Split liver transplantation – outlook to the future

When I speak about complications related to liver transplantation with a patient, I never mention the main complication of liver transplantation – being not transplanted. According to UNOS a significant number of patients on the waiting list will have to wait longer than two years, which is unacceptable. It means, depending on the indication, that many of these patients will have to die. And due to expansion of indication and shortage of organs, mortality on the waiting list continuously rises. In Europe the number of liver transplantations has plateaued for about four years now. That means we cannot expect expansion of the numbers of donors in the next few years. So the only answer to this dilemma – beyond improving the liver transplantations in our patients we perform today – is shown in Fig. 1. It is a slide in a lecture one might give in 3 to 4 years routinely showing that a donor has to give 2 lungs, 1 heart, 2 kidneys and 2 livers. For many years, anatomy has already been talking about two livers. One speaks of removing the right liver or the left liver. Yet this is not anchored enough in the mind of the liver transplant surgeon. Today we must think of the liver as source for two liver grafts as a standard concept. The donor has to be considered as one with two livers and both have to be allocated like other paired organs. As reported by Azoulay et al. (1996), de Ville de Goyet et al. (1999) and Busuttil et al. (1999), the liver is a splitable organ in about 30% of the cases. So the first step is to define the donor that is ideal for splitting. Basic characteristics for the ideal donor would be an age of less than 60 years and more than 70 kg of body weight. There should be no history of cardiac risk and the donor should be in a dynamically stable condition with no or minimal vasopressors. The liver should be free of steatosis and the presumed liver weight should be above 1.8 kg. A donor like this should be reported to the allocating organization as a donor with two livers. To minimize organizational problems due to the fact that one has to deal with two recipient centers, surgical techniques to split the liver need to be standardized. The right liver should be the one without the vena cava, with the right hepatic vein only (no middle vein) and with part of the right pedicle. There is a lot of experience with this approach especially from living-related donation as reported by Professor Tanaka.

I would propose that this part of the graft be named the Tanaka Kyoto standard. We may consider the right part of the living donor as the right liver of the split. If the right liver is accepted according to the usual rules as a graft by a recipient center, the left liver should be proposed via the sharing organization according to the same rules.

Splitting the liver for two adults is the only way to increase the graft pool. There is no competition with the living donor. The latter must be encouraged especially when time is a major issue. It will to some extent expand the donor pool; however, it will never have the impact as splitting the liver does. Finally, there will be no competition between splitting the liver and domino liver transplantation, as the latter requires a specific recipient. On that point I always have to address xenotransplantation as a solution for graft shortage. Today we do not have any realistic approach to graft the liver from a different species. Maybe in the far, far future research will develop methods to make the xenotransplantation possible.

Coming to the end of my talk – I do not want to talk about the future, because – I think – the future is today. Many technical problems have been solved. We are able to define the donor eligible for split liver transplantation. We have found ways to organize the distribution of two liver grafts of one donor. We really should now go all the way! I would like to close this lecture by reminding you that the liver has not two parts, but incorporates eight segments.

GPSR Compliance

The European Union's (EU) General Product Safety Regulation (GPSR) is a set of rules that requires consumer products to be safe and our obligations to ensure this.

If you have any concerns about our products, you can contact us on ProductSafety@springernature.com

In case Publisher is established outside the EU, the EU authorized representative is:

Springer Nature Customer Service Center GmbH
Europaplatz 3
69115 Heidelberg, Germany

Batch number: 10725973

Printed by Printforce, the Netherlands